MY PERIOD POWER!

Period Confidence Guide:
For Girls
Tweens, Teens & Young Adults
Ultimate Period Positivity Toolkit!

Conquer the Fear and Gear of Puberty, Hormones, Emotions and First Menstruation

Part of the **MY POWER!** Series
Book 2

♥♥

SheriBelle Karper

Kingman Publications LLC

ISBN: 978-1-967750-02-3 (paperback) • LCCN: 2025910285 (paperback)

ISBN: 978-1-967750-03-0 (ebook)

ISBN: 978-1-967750-14-6 (hardback)

ISBN: 978-1-967750-19-1 (audiobook)

Printed in the United States of America

1st Edition ©2025

Ultimate Empowerment Book for Puberty and Period Positivity

MY PERIOD POWER!

Period Confidence Guide

For Girls
Tweens, Teens and Young Adults

By SheriBelle Karper

FOR GIRLS

Conquer the Fear and Gear of First Menstruation

KINGMAN PUBLICATIONS

Contents

Foreword by Dr. Renee Cotter, MD, OB/GYN, FACOG

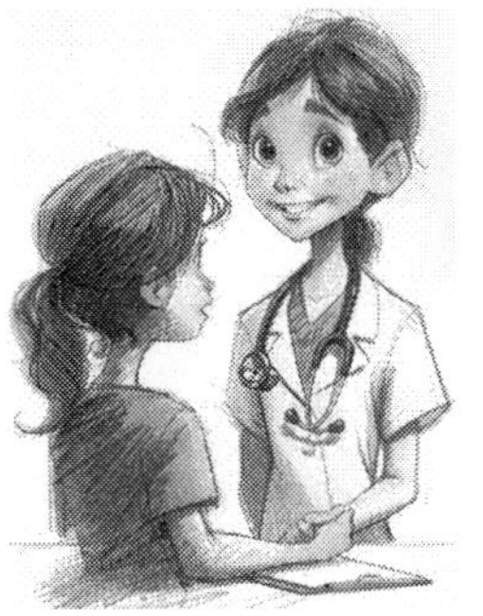

As an obstetrician and gynecologist with over 30 years of experience in Southern California, I have dedicated my career to supporting women through the various stages of their lives. From the early years of puberty to the complexities of menopause, I have witnessed the profound physical and emotional changes that define womanhood. It is from this perspective that I wholeheartedly endorse SheriBelle Karper's invaluable guides *MY PERIOD POWER!, MY SOCIAL POWER!* and *MY BODY POWER!*

These books offer not just information, but a compassionate roadmap through the often daunting journey of puberty. SheriBelle masterfully navigates the physical transformations and the emotional landscapes that accompany this pivotal time, providing practical advice and heartfelt encouragement to help young adults embrace their evolving identities.

In *MY SOCIAL POWER!*, SheriBelle goes beyond the basics of physical care; she addresses the emotional and social challenges that can arise during this tumultuous period. Her insights into navigating social media and making safe choices are particularly relevant in today's digital age, where young teens face pressures that many of us from earlier generations can hardly imagine. By using language that resonates with young readers, SheriBelle ensures that her messages are not only accessible but also engaging.

Reflecting on my own experiences, I realize how fortunate I am to have grown up in a time without the influence of social media. After reading *MY BODY POWER!*, I realize again that conversations about menstruation or sexuality were often hushed, leaving many of us to navigate these changes in silence. *MY PERIOD POWER!* reminds me of the awkward moment of telling my mother I had started my period, only to receive a brief response about where to find pads. This lack of open dialogue fueled my passion for women's health and highlighted the necessity for clear, supportive resources.

MY PERIOD POWER!, MY SOCIAL POWER! and *MY BODY POWER!* are essential tools for young adults and should be seen as vital references for parents, educators, and healthcare professionals alike. They empower young readers to not only understand their bodies but to celebrate them. I envision a future where every young teen receives a copy of these books as a rite of passage, guiding them through the challenges of puberty with confidence and grace.

I encourage everyone who cares for or mentors young teens to embrace SheriBelle's work. Together, we can foster a generation of informed, empowered young adults who love themselves and their bodies.

Dr. Renee Cotter, MD, OB/GYN, FACOG

Dedication

To My Parents…
Thank you for the gift of curiosity.

♥

To my pre-period self…
Don't worry about it. It's all going to be fine.

♥

To my family…
I know I drove you crazy, so thank you for sticking with me.

Epigraph

A girl should be two things: who and what she wants.
— Coco Chanel

Be yourself; everyone else is already taken.
— Oscar Wilde

I believe in being strong when everything seems to be going wrong. I believe that happy girls are the prettiest girls. I believe that tomorrow is another day, and I believe in miracles.
— Audrey Hepburn

The trick is growing up without growing old.
— Casey Stengel

1. Hey! I've Been Waiting for You!

Yayyyyyyy! You made it!

Welcome to ***MY PERIOD POWER!***—your all-in-one book, your go-to guide for all the fantastic, weird, and powerful changes happening in your body. One minute you're just living your life, and the next, your body is doing things you never signed up for, like getting taller, curvier, sprouting hair (yes, even *there*), a period, and throwing your emotions on a rollercoaster with no seatbelt. Fun, right?

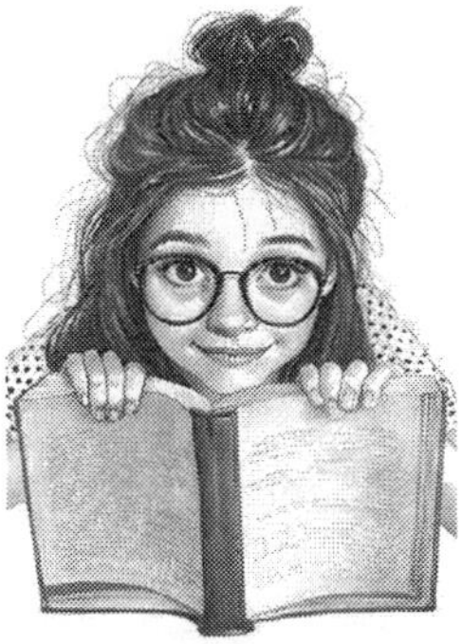

And then—Boom!—you have to deal with people who either act like periods are disgusting, guys who have no idea what's going on, and a world that sometimes treats this totally normal period thing like it's a bad secret. You're probably asking yourself, "Are you kidding me?"

Or have you ever just found yourself lying in bed, staring at the ceiling, wondering what it's going to be like to grow up? Like… Will you live in a castle? Will you have a pet dragon? Will you have kids? Or maybe just a fridge full of snacks that no one else touches?

Growing up can feel like this mystery wrapped and glitter and weirdness. One day, you're climbing trees and making slime, and the next—Boom!—your body's like, "Surprise! We're becoming an adult now!" (Umm, excuse me?!)

But don't worry—this book is like your older, cooler cousin, who tells you all the good stuff without being awkward about it. We're going to talk about all the changes (yes, even *those* changes), what they mean, and how to handle them like the confident human you are.

So if you've ever wondered *what the heck is happening with my body??*—You're in the right place!

This Book? It's Different

Let's get one thing straight: This is NOT your typical book. No boring, scientific lectures here. Nope. No catching Zzz's in this book. This is like your cool, slightly quirky guide to understanding and conquering your period. We are looking at the good, the bad, and the kind of icky parts of menstruation.

This is us, chatting like besties about what's happening to your body and how to handle it like a pro. There will be slang, jokes, and a whole lot of keeping it real. We're talking body confidence, period hacks, and all the things nobody tells you. And trust me, the more you understand, the easier this whole growing up thing gets. Win-Win!

And just so you know, you are NOT alone in this. Every single girl who has ever lived has gone through these changes. I did...your mother did... and even your grandma (Yes, even her!). So if you feel overwhelmed or totally confused, that's OK. Growing up comes with big changes, but let me tell you, you're exactly where you were supposed to be right now.

I Won't Talk Down To You

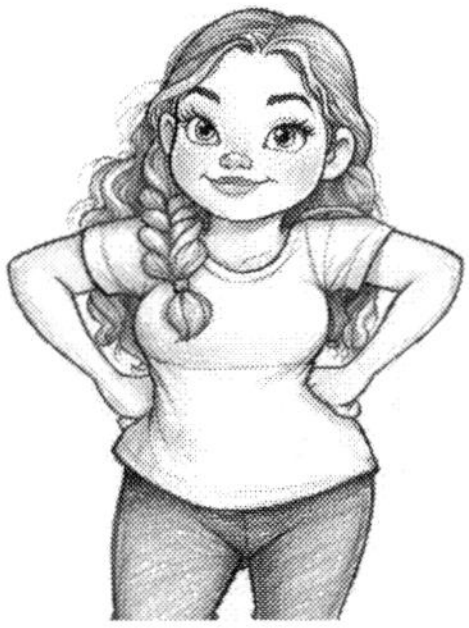

My agreement with you: I want you to know that I see you for the incredible person you are becoming, not a little kid but a tween or a teen who is now stepping into your adult power, so I'm going to talk to you that way. There will not be any "little kid" talk because that's not who you are.

With all this change, you might feel a little different on the inside, too. You might be feeling more pumped, more irritable, or maybe more nervous about stuff than before. Yeah, that's also completely okay, and it's simply another part of growing up.

What's Inside?

Here's what we're going to tackle together:

- **First, we'll dive into the changes** happening in your body and talk about how to embrace them with confidence, even when you feel awkward or weird.
- **Next, we'll break down everything** you need to know about periods: Why they happen, how to handle them, the tools that you will need, and how to make them a little less overwhelming. We're cutting through the science doo-dah to tell you why your body's doing its thing every month and what's up with all the new (and sometimes weird) symptoms. (Hint: Period kits are your new BFF, btw!).
- We'll talk about all the gear: **From pads to tampons to menstrual cups.** Yup, we're doing it!
- **Then, we'll tackle how to deal with the people in your life,** especially when they don't understand what you're going through. Yes, we'll be looking at the guys on this one.

- **Finally, we'll explore how periods are viewed around the world.** Some cultures celebrate them; others still treat them like a big taboo. The more we understand, the more empowered we can be about our own experiences.
- **Feeling All the Feels?** "That time of the month" can make you feel a little emotional. We'll chat about how to keep your cool and who you can rant to when you need to.
- **Mood Swings Got You on a Wild Ride?** We are going to master the art of these emotional ninja moves together. I'll show you how to handle those emotions like a pro.
- **Yikes! Leaks at School:** Or, frankly, anywhere? Yup, we're talking about that, too.
- **Cramps Cramping Your Style?** We've got tips and tricks to kick those cramps to the curb. Are you ready to battle them like a boss? *Check!* We've got all the details on how to show them who's actually in charge.
- **When to Call in the Doctor:** Yes, sometimes we need to bring in the big guns to fight these period battles. But hey, isn't it good to know that other people are out there to help you with real answers to your specific questions and issues?
- **Your Future Self:** The power your hormones have to preserve your beauty, strength, and vitality later in life.
- **Plus, a lot more!**

By the end of this book, you'll have everything you need to own your power, love your body, and crush this whole growing up thing.

Are You Ready to Unlock Your Power?

This book is about helping you step into your boldest, most confident self. Because confidence isn't about being perfect, it's about showing up for yourself, embracing who you are, and knowing that you are already enough.

Introducing: The multi-book MY POWER! Series of Confidence and Success!

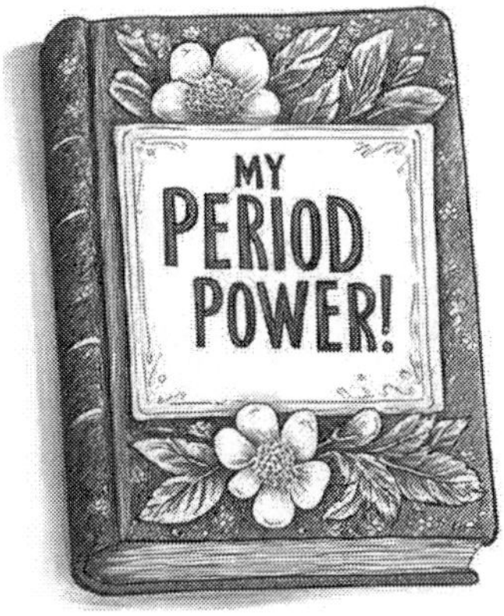

Meet Your Other BFFs: The Companion Books! If you love ***MY PERIOD POWER!:***

You'll also want to buy the companion book called ***MY BODY POWER!*** (For Girl Tweens, Teens, and Young Adults). It's a BODY CONFIDENCE GUIDE where you'll find answers to help you get to know and love your super special transforming body and how to be proud of it in this fast-changing world.

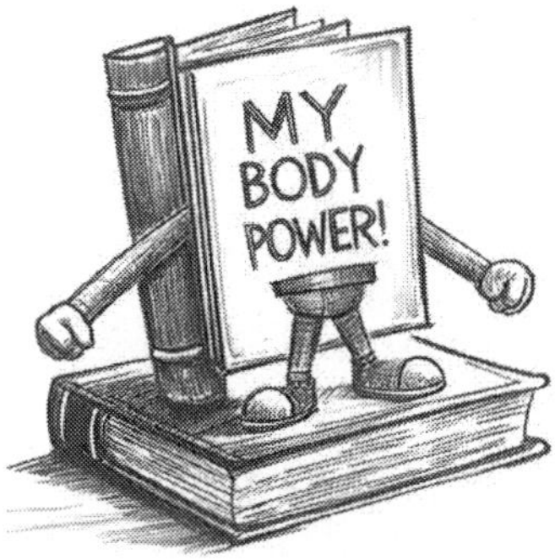

You'll want to get ***MY SOCIAL POWER!*** (For Boy & Girl Tweens, Teens, and Young Adults). It's your go-to SOCIAL CONFIDENCE GUIDE, full of tips and tricks to help you figure out your super unique and always evolving thoughts and group interactions. It's about learning how to handle social situations like a pro, feeling good about yourself, and owning your vibe no matter what's happening around you in this wild, fast-moving world. Let's crush it together!

Soon, there will be the ***MY PERIOD POWER! WORKBOOK*** (For Girl Tweens, Teens, and Young Adults), where you can journal, predict your period schedule, and monitor your moods, along with fun puzzles, recipes, and beautiful coloring pages. It will also be available where you got this book. Fun!

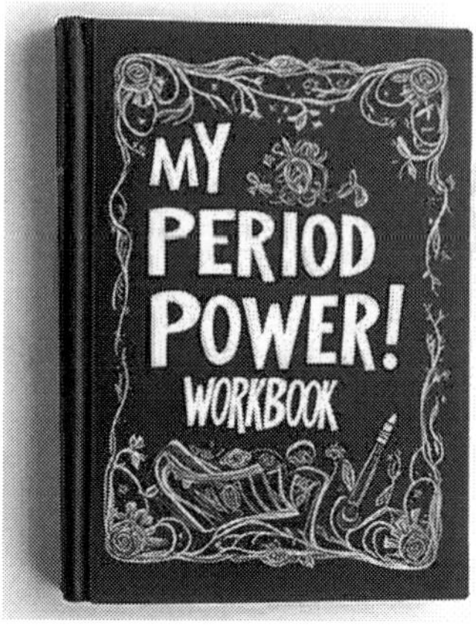

And, also the ***MY SOCIAL POWER! WORKBOOK*** (For Boy & Girl Tweens, Teens, and Young Adults) which will contain journaling, goal-setting, gratitude listing, prompts for writing, and other great things! This too will also be available where you got this book.

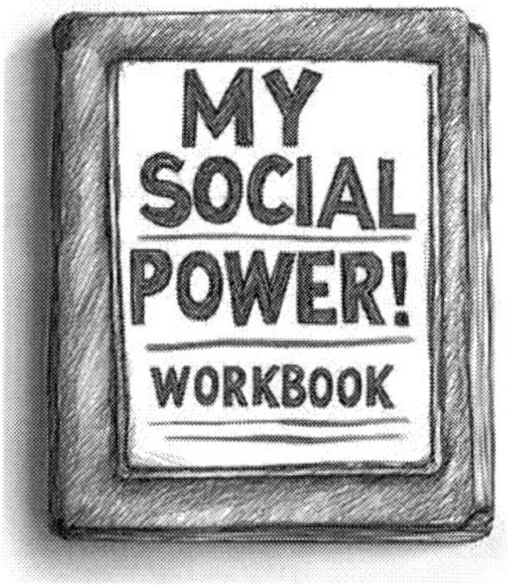

This book contains the word "girl" and other feminine terms because I think that's who will probably read it. But hey, if that word doesn't fit with who you are, swap it out for a word that fits you better. That way, you will still get all the awesome info in this book.

By the time you flip the last page of this book, you will be a total pro when it comes to your period. You'll know all the ins and outs, the ups and the downs, and all the hocus-pocus that seems like magic now, but instead, you'll know the science behind it. (Eeeek!) Please don't be nervous, it's really cool stuff!

You'll know what's happening and why it's happening. It's like you'll become a period expert and share that knowledge with your friends. It will give you the confidence to handle whatever comes your way. Pretty cool, right?

So, Who Am I?

So let me introduce myself! I'm SheriBelle Karper, and I guess you could say that my entire life has been about confidence. Please make sure you take a look at the **About The Author** section at the back of the book. I think you'll be a little impressed by all the things I've done in my life! I tell you these things because they are all things *YOU* can do in your life, too. It all depends on your choices and what's important to you.

Anything is possible… or impossible… it all depends on how you look at life. I personally like the word *possible* much more than *impossible.* "Possible" gets you places. "Impossible" keeps you stuck.

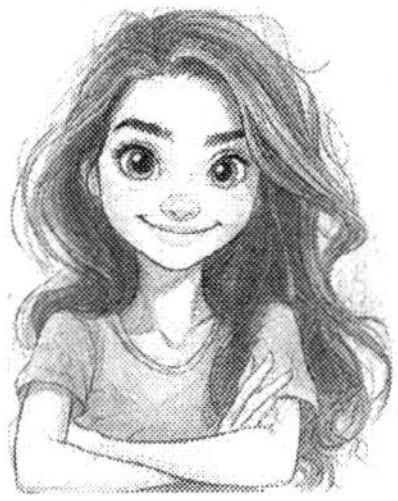

All the experiences that are written about me in my **About The Author** chapter have shaped the way I see the world; the way I see confidence and the way I see what is "possible." To me, confidence isn't about having all the answers. It's about showing up for yourself, trying new things, and embracing who you are, even when it feels a little scary. It's about celebrating your quirks, learning from your mistakes, and being brave enough to take on the world one step at a time. And I promise, you already have everything you need to do that, you just might not see it yet. Yes, everything is "possible."

That's exactly why I hope to inspire you with ***MY PERIOD POWER!*** It's a book filled with stories, advice, and tips to help you find your own strength and voice during this exciting and sometimes overwhelming time in your life.

My mission is to help you discover your own power and potential. If I've learned one thing from all my adventures, it's that the greatest journey you'll ever take is the one about believing in yourself. And trust me, you've got what it takes. You were actually born with everything you need. You just need to learn how to find it.

Also, make sure you check out the amazing **Foreword written by Dr. Renee Cotter, OB/GYN, FACOG!** I feel so honored that she wanted to be a part of this book, and she made this plainly clear in her phenomenal foreward. She's a very popular gynecologist and obstetrician for over 30 years in Los Angeles, California. So please, go ahead and check it out!

After reading this book, you will feel even more confident about your changing body and what you can accomplish during your period. Imagine feeling totally in charge of all the changes happening inside you and rocking it! (Yeah!) That's what we're aiming for. You'll understand so much that you'll feel stronger and more confident every single day!

It's Good to Talk About These Things

There might be times when something in this book has you asking questions, or you're super curious and want to dig deeper. That's totally fine. Frankly, I encourage it. It's super important to talk about all of it. If you've got questions or something doesn't click, chat about it with your parents or maybe a teacher. Please make sure it's someone you and your family really trust.

Okay, gorgeous, you're already bright and beautiful and pretty darn amazing just as you are, but it's about time we get started on this big discovery called your period!

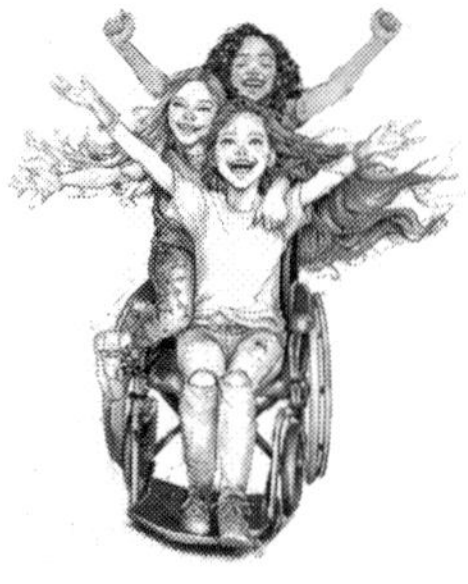

After reading this book, you will feel even more confident about your changing body and what you can accomplish during your period. Imagine feeling totally in charge of all the changes happening inside you and rocking it! (Yeah!) That's what we're aiming for.

Getting the hang of your period is like unlocking a superpower. Seriously, it might seem overwhelming at first, but as soon as you master this stuff, you'll feel unstoppable.

Grab a cozy spot, keep an open mind, and get ready to discover how awesome your body truly is! This is your journey, and I'm here to cheer you on every step of the way. Let's get started—your period power is waiting!

Ready to conquer the world? Let's goooooo... It's game time!

ACTION TAKEAWAYS:

- This is not your average book. It's written like how people talk to each other in a conversation.
- Change is good, but sometimes change is not always easy.
- Get ***MY BODY POWER!*** (For Girl Tweens, Teens, and Young Adults), ***MY SOCIAL POWER!*** (For Boy & Girl Tweens, Teens, and Young Adults), and the ***MY SOCIAL POWER! WORKBOOK*** (For Boy & Girl Tweens, Teens, and Young Adults) along with the ***MY PERIOD POWER! WORKBOOK*** (For Girl Tweens, Teens, and Young Adults) to help you through these big changes in your life.
- Ask questions and find answers. Listen closely and use that great advice.

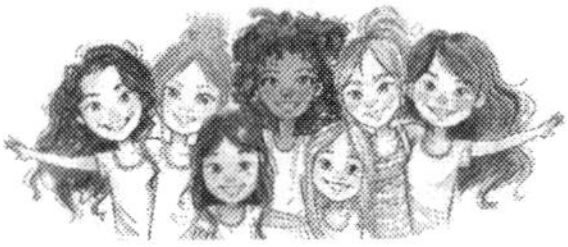

2. My Period Power!

Why This Book is Going to Be Your New BFF!

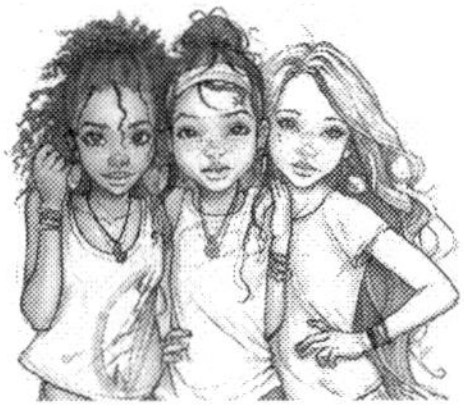

You've probably picked up ***MY PERIOD POWER!*** thinking, *Finally, somebody gets it!* —and trust me, I do! But then again, since we've only just met, you might think, "What the heck is this?! My period power? Period? What?"

Just know that things will come into focus pretty soon. It's completely fine that you're wondering what's going on and that you're totally new to this. In fact, in some ways, it's better because your mind isn't full of gossipy blah-blah that might not be exactly true.

And guess what? Every person who has had their period was totally new to this at some point in their lives. So, no problem! You're right on time! And shortly, you're going to be turning that, "Hey wait, I'm new to this," into "Hey, I've got this period thing DOWN!"

Come On, Give Me a Hint!

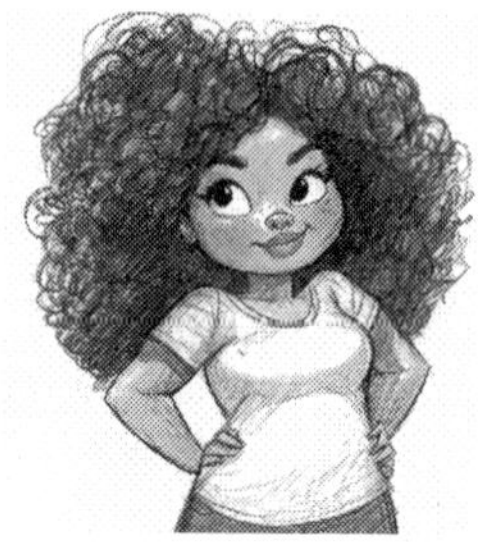

It's simple: Your body is throwing you a monthly party, and you're the guest of honor. This book is your party planner, getting you ready with all the info.

And who is the mastermind behind getting you this book? Probably your mom, dad, teacher, or maybe an older sibling who's already been to the party and knows the drill. They've seen the signs coming from you; signs you didn't even know you were showing. Maybe you've been dealing with mood swings, food cravings, or maybe a sudden interest in chocolate! Hahaha! Yup! Those are the signs that you're going through puberty and that your period is coming.

Why did they get you this book? They want to help you deal with the ups and downs of growing up and having your period without feeling like you're on a never-ending mystery tour. They probably want to also avoid the awkward questions and give you the lowdown in a way that's totally chill, not embarrassing, and not a total bore-fest. Now you've got this book to guide you through it, and we're going to have a giggle or two along the way, I promise!

Talking about puberty is an excellent way to begin a real conversation with your parents. You'll probably each share amazing stories about growing up. Some will be hysterical, while others might make you a little teary-eyed. But, I guarantee that as you have these talks, your relationship will bloom into something that strengthens and deepens your connection. It could really be an incredible moment.

There's something about sharing stories with someone you care about —it's deep and it's amazing!

BONUS PRO TIP:

You should have the people who got you this book also get themselves a copy of ***MY PERIOD POWER!*** Then you can all read the book at the same time. That way, when you have questions or things you want to discuss (and you will), you can make notes and mark the sections to do that. Plus, keep your eye out for the ***MY PERIOD POWER! WORKBOOK*** for tracking and journaling your period. It will also have fun puzzles, jokes, recipes, and beautiful coloring pages.

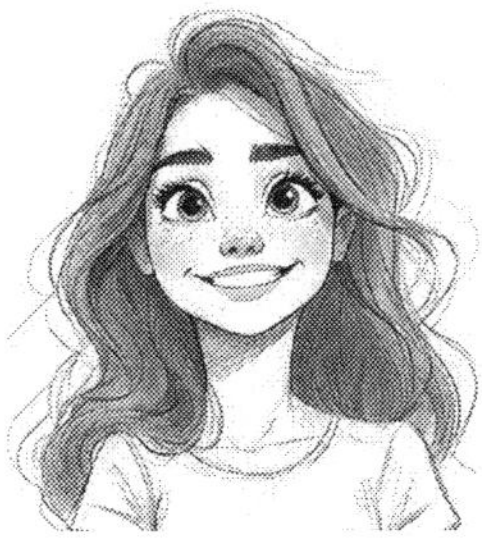

Let's Talk About Periods (For Real)

Yeah, we're going there. No whispering, no code words, just straight talk about that time of the month. ***MY PERIOD POWER!*** is here to spill all the tea on periods, why they can sometimes be a total pain, and why they are kind of amazing (yes, really!). We're discovering why they happen, how to deal with them, and how to not let them ruin your day (or your favorite pair of jeans).

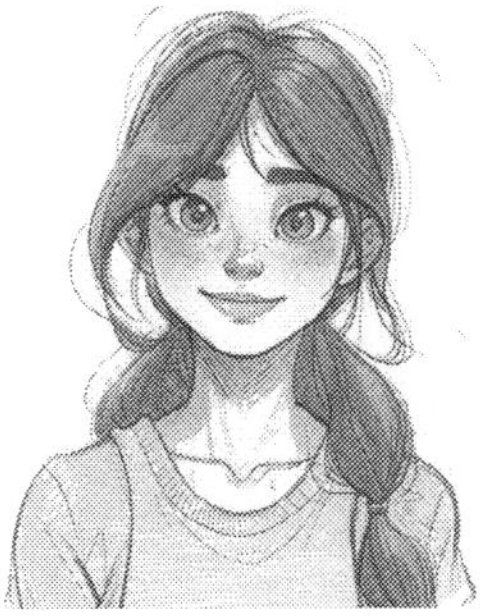

What Is This Period Thing *Exactly*?

Wow! You want to get right into it, eh? I admire that. I really do! Okay, Hermione, it's time for some magic and the big reveal…

Basically, your period is something that happens to girls as they grow up. It usually starts around your age or a bit older. Every month, the body gets ready for a possible baby by making the inside of your tummy super soft and cozy (specifics coming later). The body doesn't need that cozy stuff if there's no baby, so it exits out near where you pee, and this is what we call your period.

So, what comes out? It's mostly blood, but don't get nervous. It's totally normal and part of how your body works. That's the short version. A little weird? Yeah. There will be more details later, but yeah, in the beginning, it seems a little weird.

But here's a surprise: You've just stumbled upon your secret weapon in the battle against the period blues. Welcome to the club! ***MY PERIOD POWER!*** will become your period playbook, your monthly mantra, and your go-to manual for turning those "Why me?" moments into "Hey, I've got this!" victories.

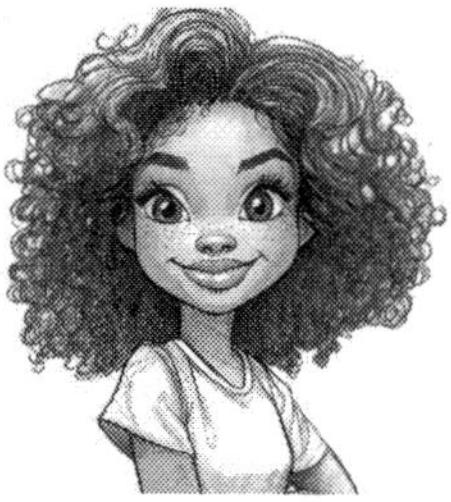

I'll be sharing the real deal about what's happening inside you, cool stories from people just like you, and some genius ways to handle all the period drama.

You're going through a lot of change right now, and if there's one thing I can guarantee you, you'll be going through a lot more. So, it's the perfect time to learn how to roll with all these changes.

<u>**IMPORTANT:**</u>

I know I'm using playful language in this book. It's just like you and I are having a real face-to-face conversation. I'm doing that because it makes it fun and easy to read. But please, make no mistake, these are real concerns with real skills about growing up to help you tackle all of these things you will face soon or are facing right now.

Sometimes some of these changes are going to make you a little emotional. I understand, I've been there. I want you to know that all the emotions that you're feeling during this time are real and valid.

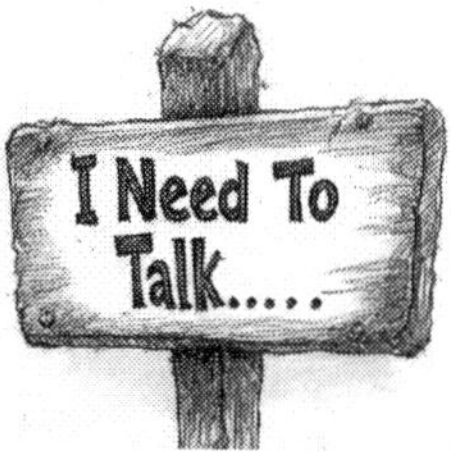

PLUS, including your special support crew (like your parents) in the discussion, will help you make the right decisions.

Because trust me… there will be decisions.

You can look at this book, but you also will need their advice. This is a group effort. We cannot do this growing-up thing alone without the support and love of our most treasured people.

It's important that you tell them, "Hey, I need to talk about ____________" (fill in the blank). Make sure they've heard you correctly, and then make sure you do your part to be a good listener. Have a back-and-forth conversation so that everything gets said and everything gets heard, but mostly, to get the answers you need.

BONUS PRO TIP:

You can jump around this book if you like. Do you see a chapter that is important to you right now? Then read it! Mark it with a "Check" mark, then come back and pick up where you left off. Try to read the entire book.

MY PERIOD POWER!

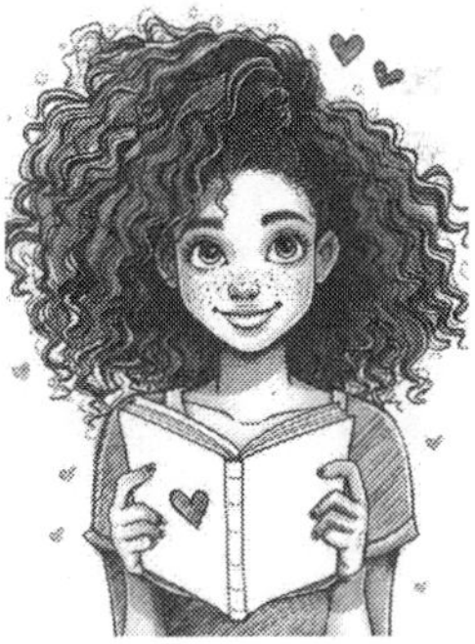

By the end of this book, you won't just be surviving your period, you'll be thriving! So, whether you're reading this hiding under your covers, or laughing with your friends, let's kick those period blues away together. You won't just be getting by when *Aunt Flo* comes to visit, you'll be throwing out the welcome mat and saying, "Let's do this."

You might not exactly be marking your calendar with hearts and smiley faces for your next period, but you definitely won't be *freaking out* about it, and you'll see that your period isn't as bad as you thought. In fact, you could find yourself looking forward to it. Okay, maybe you won't be looking forward to it, but you definitely won't be *dreading* it. And, if we are feeling the blues (I mean, really feeling them), then we should be kind to ourselves and reach out to others for the support we need.

Ready Freddie? So, here's to you, Period Posse, our new tribe! Where we turn "My Period, Ugh!" into "My Period Rocks!" (Or at least, "My period isn't that bad, actually.")

Let's Do This! Let the Journey Begin!

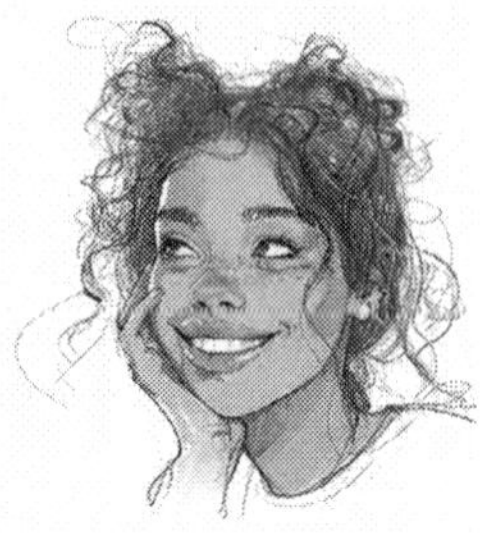

ACTION TAKEAWAYS:

- It's okay to feel all the feels. Your body and mind are changing rapidly right now, and sometimes it takes some getting used to.
- Buy the companion books to help you on your journey.

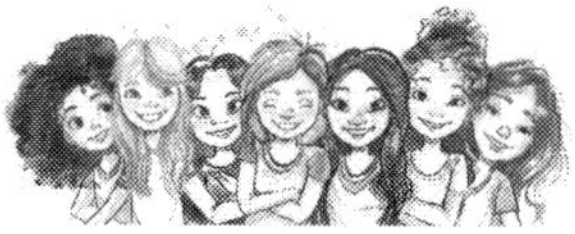

3. Which Came First? The Hormone or the Egg?

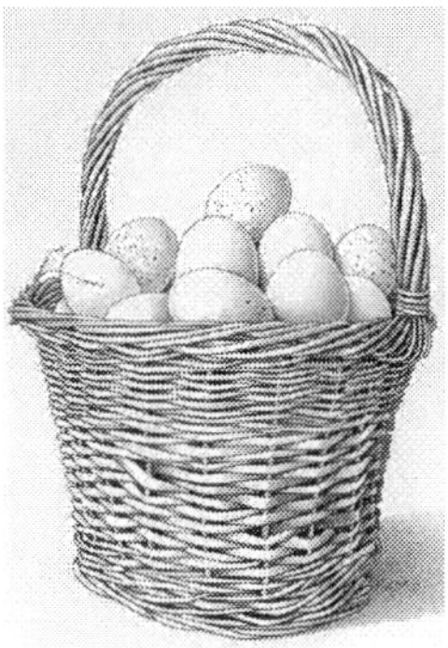

Whoa, dudette! That's deep! I didn't realize you were so profound! Great question, by the way. Okay then, let's get started!

A Brief History of Your Body From the Beginning

All right, think of it this way: When a baby girl is still growing inside her mom, her body sets up hormones and future egg cells almost at the same time. Her body is getting ready for the big party that won't happen until she's much older, like when she hits puberty.

- **Egg Cells (Eggs):** These special cells are the VIP guests for a party planned for far in the future. Every girl is born with all the egg cells she will ever have. They're just hanging out, not doing much, waiting for this gigantic event—puberty. This is when the body says, "Okay, it might be time to get one of these VIPs ready each month." But remember, these VIP guests were on the guest list from the very start, even before a girl was born.

- **Hormones:** These are the signals or messages that run everything, telling different parts of your body what to do and when. They're like the party planners and messengers. Some hormones are around doing basic jobs, even when a girl is just a baby. But the major work, like causing periods to start and making it possible for you to have a baby, doesn't kick off until puberty. That's when the hormones really start ramping up their activity, getting everything ready for the monthly party where an egg gets the spotlight and says, "Time to party!"

If you're asking who showed up first (the hormone or the egg), it's kind of a tie. The egg cells and the stuff needed to make hormones get ready at about the same time a girl is still a tiny baby inside her mom. But they both wait until the moment is right (puberty) to begin their main jobs.

Okay, the history lesson is o-ver!

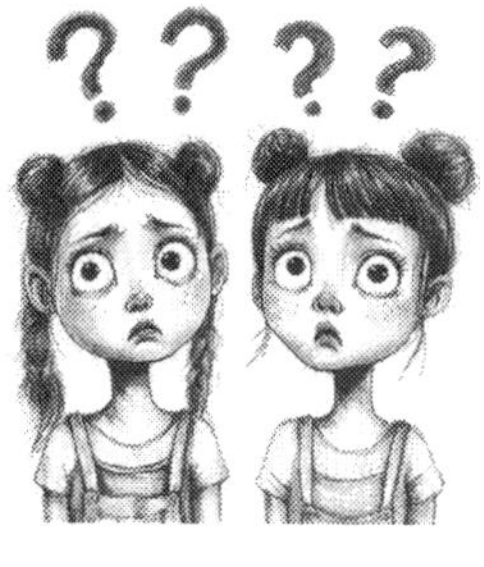

What's Up With Puberty and That First Period?

Puberty seems like it's this crazy carnival ride your body decides to ride without asking you first. One day, you're chilling, and the next, you've got boobs growing, hair sprouting in weird places, and yeah, that thing called a period.

Puberty is the time when your body starts changing from a kid's body into an adult's. You grow taller, your body changes shape, you get curvier, you might get zits, and you feel moodier than usual. Does any of this sound familiar to you? If so, CONGRATULATIONS! You're probably going through puberty right now, and that's the reason you got this book!

Puberty is a curious thing, and everyone's body and mind react differently. It can start pretty early for some girls, like 8 or 9 years old, but can even be as late as 16. That's a huge age range, but no age is better or worse, just different. Just because you may start early or late doesn't make it better or worse; it just makes it different from the next girl.

Understanding Puberty, Your Body and Your Period

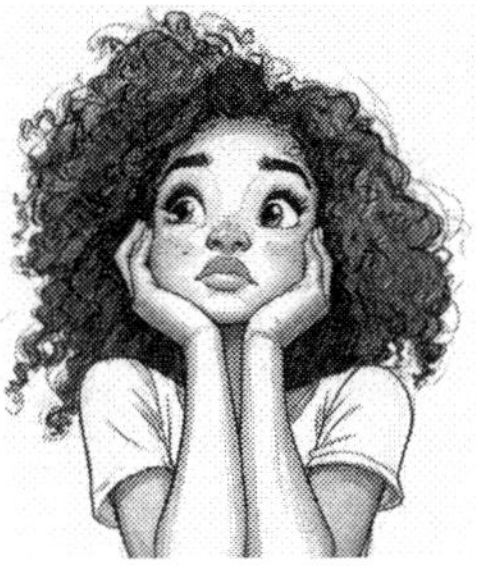

Puberty is basically your body's way of saying, "Hey, you're starting to hit that time where you can make babies." But since that's probably not on your to-do list right now, let's focus on what's really going on. You'll get all these signals from your brain to produce hormones. They are like text messages that tell your body to kick things into a higher gear.

It doesn't matter what body type you are, puberty will find you. Puberty is all about change, and your body is changing a lot right now. Whether you are tall, short, lean, or curvy, your body is perfect for you, and I'm even going so far as to say—It's beautiful! You can even go into the bathroom right now, look in the mirror and say (or scream!) "I'M BEAUTIFUL!" Heehee! I love it! Yeah, go ahead, I'll wait!

If you have any doubts about the incredibleness of your body, get those thoughts out of your head right now! Your body is an incredible masterpiece! If you give it food, rest, and a little love, it will last you many, many years. Sure, every once in a while we need to take it into the mechanic, but mostly, it's a finely tuned machine that literally billions of people have test-driven over many centuries!

Puberty includes breast development (Eeeek!), hair growth (like in really weird places! (Whaaat?!)), and you guessed it—your first period (Wooow!). It's like a monthly memo saying everything is working as it should. It might feel weird and sometimes totally unfair since guys don't have a period, but keep in mind, guys will never be able to have a baby, and that's incredibly special. But trust me, it's all part of the awesome (okay, sometimes annoying) process of growing up.

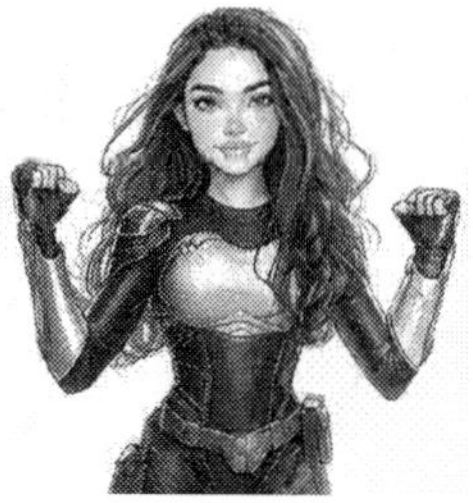

The Science of Menstruation (Seriously, It's Not Rocket Science)

Here's the lowdown on why we get periods. Like I said, most girls get their period around age 13, but it can happen as early as 8 years old and even up to 16.

Inside your belly, you've got these two things called ovaries. They're like tiny egg factories. Every month, they drop an egg, and your system says, "Let's get this place ready in case we're having a baby!" That's when the walls of your uterus get all cozy and soft.

But when no baby shows up, your body says, "Okay, party's over," and it gets rid of all that cozy stuff. That's what "menstruation" is. It cleans house and makes everything fresh again. It's a little yucky and can sometimes be a pain (literally), but it's your body doing its natural thing, making sure that everything is working A-OK.

We've covered the basics of why periods happen, but let's go a bit deeper into what's actually going on each month. Your menstrual cycle isn't just about that one week of *period blood.* It's a process that starts on the first day of your period and keeps rolling until the first day of your next period.

The whole "cycle" lasts about a month—one week with your period, then three weeks without. It's your very own monthly subscription, except you didn't sign up for it, and you can't cancel it (bummer, I know). It can vary by a couple of days here and there, especially in the beginning. But when you get older, your periods will probably become pretty regular and you can pretty much anticipate exactly when your period will start.

In every cycle, your hormones are going up and down. They are behind the scenes, making sure the egg cell gets released (ovulation) and then telling your uterus to get ready just in case a baby starts growing. It's a lot of work your female parts are doing each month.

No baby? No problem! Your body just hits the reset button (a.k.a. your period), and the whole cycle starts over.

Dealing With Those Crazy Period Symptoms

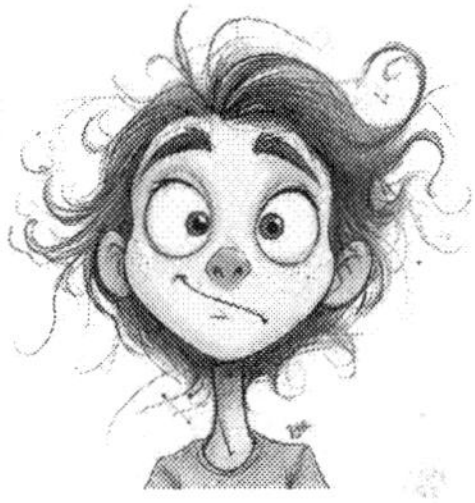

Now, let's talk about the things that can make your period a little difficult. Cramps, for starters. They range from "Oh, that's annoying" to "Why, oh why, can't I just stay in bed all day?" Cramps happen because your uterus is contracting (basically squeezing its muscles) to help shed this monthly lining. Imagine, it's like your uterus is doing Olympic-level gymnastics inside your tummy. Sometimes, it's not so fun.

Then there are the mood swings. One minute you're laughing, and the next you're crying because your sock won't go on right. It's all thanks to those wild hormone ups and downs. Let's not forget the cravings—chocolate, potato chips, you name it. It's like your body thinks it's going to a deserted island and needs all the snacks NOW!

First Period Stories (Because They Never Get Old, Haha!)

Everybody's got their own unique story about their first period. Some might be chilling at home, some might start at school, and some might start at the worst possible moment, like right before a pool party. And the reactions? It can be "Ew, what is happening?" to "Yes! Finally, I'm not a kid anymore!"

- Jesse said "I thought I was dying when I first saw my period blood!"

- And then there's Alex, who was so prepared (thanks to her older sister), she practically threw a party.
- Or my neighbor, Zoe, who thought she'd get her period in the middle of class and wore pads to school every day for a whole year. When it finally happened, she said, "That's it? I've been wearing these things for nothing?"
- My own personal story: Let's just say, I wasn't excited about becoming a member of the period club right before I had to go to ballet class. Having to wear pink tights and a leotard. (Aaaaargh!) I wanted my period to start for so long because all my friends already had their periods. But when the moment finally came, I thought I was going to faint! I saw stars! The room was spinning. I had to sit down. Is this really happening? I called my mom, and she started crying, so happy that I was becoming a woman. "Ugh, thanks Mom." *Click.*

My point here is that everybody's experience is different. Every girl's first period (called menarche) is like a badge of honor, so how each person reacts to it will be different. There is no right or wrong answer. You do you, baby! Be proud!

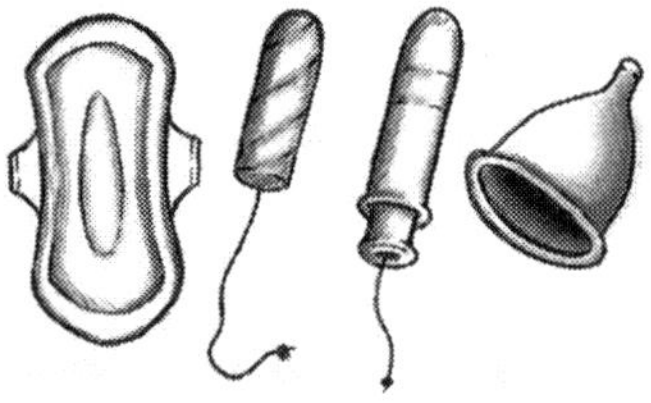

No matter how it happens, just know you're not alone. Every girl has been there or will be at some point. And this book? It's here to make sure you're smiling, learning, and ready to tackle that period head-on.

Your Period Product Cheat Sheet

Pads, tampons, menstrual cups—oh my! We'll touch more on this later, but choosing what to use can feel like trying to pick a favorite ice cream flavor—there are several options. Pads are like the comfy sweats of period products; no fuss, just stick them in your undies and go. Tampons? They're sort of like skinny jeans. They take a bit of time to get used to, but are great for swimming or running. And menstrual cups are like those high-tech sneakers. They're sort of intimidating at first, but once you get the hang of them, they're game changers.

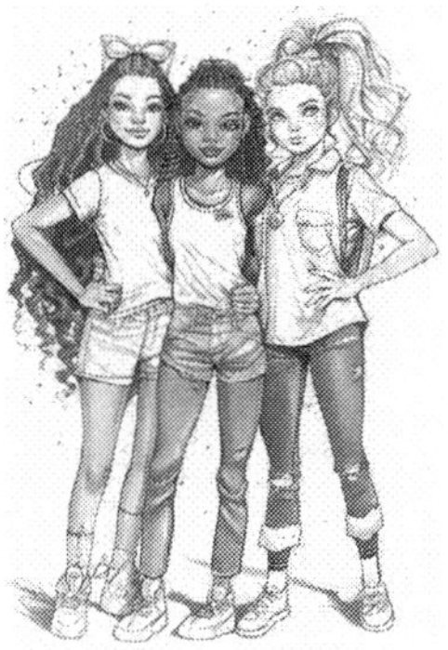

You've Got This!

Here's the thing: Your periods might seem like the worst thing ever, especially when you're trying to figure out how to take some control over them. But you need to listen to me here—you're stronger than you think you are. Together, with this book, we're going to tackle all the weird, awkward, and, yes, even the cool parts of having a period. You and me together, we've got this!

And who knows? By the end of ***MY PERIOD POWER!***, ***MY BODY POWER!***, and ***MY PERIOD POWER! WORKBOOK,*** you'll be armed with all the knowledge, tips, and tricks to deal with your period like a boss.

ACTION TAKEAWAYS:

- Eggs and hormones are inside you from the very beginning.
- Go to the store or look online and start to take a peek at pads, tampons, and menstrual cups—the players we're going to be dealing with.
- Talk about these things with your parents or a trusted adult to get the answers to your questions.

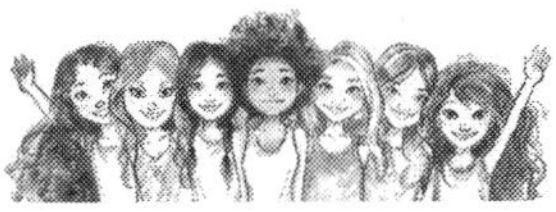

4. But I Kind Of Still Want To Be a Kid...

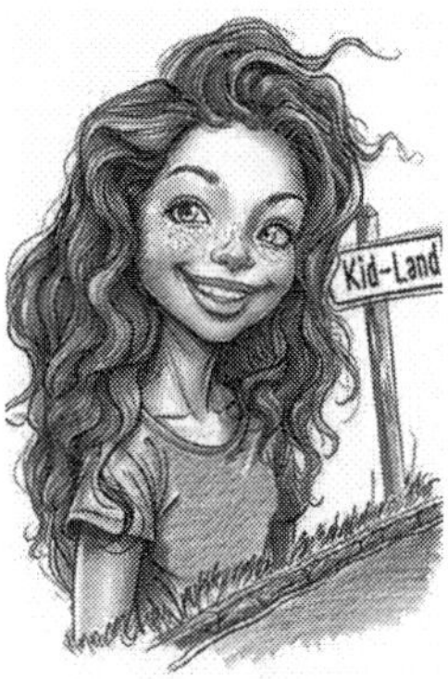

I totally get it. One minute, you're ruling the schoolyard at four square, and the next minute —Wham!—your period starts, and it feels like everyone expects you to act grown-up overnight.

Newsflash: It's not really like that, but yeah, it kind of feels like a mega jump from kid-mode straight into adulthood.

When you get your period for the first time, it can feel like you're being fast-forwarded into being a grown-up. Like suddenly, you're supposed to understand all this adult stuff. You like the idea of growing up, but a period? That wasn't in the plan, was it? And honestly, you just want to smack that pause button and stay in Kidville a little longer. You're not the only one. I felt that way, too. It's totally normal.

I know, I know, hearing something is normal doesn't fix it, but it just lets you know that you're not an alien. You're a real human being going through real human things, and you need to hear it. You need to hear that you are normal.

The Struggle Is Real

Feeling rushed? It might seem like getting your period is your one-way ticket out of your sweet childhood, but no, it's really just a heads up that things are changing, and you're about to start some awesome new adventures in this thing called life.

So, take a deep breath. Yeah, I mean right now. Take a deep breath, I'll wait…

And repeat after me, "Nobody learns everything all at once… like, ever."

Do remember your first soccer game? You didn't just storm the field knowing all the plays, right? Nope. It took time to figure out how to kick the ball and learn all the rules and skills (a lot of time, right?). Period stuff is the same deal. Getting used to the idea and figuring it all out will take time.

Changes Can Be Weird

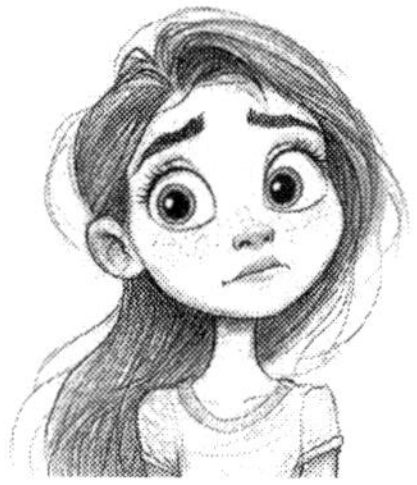

Your body is changing, and it can feel a little strange. I mean, you just got hit with the *blood* talk, and usually, blood is not our favorite topic unless we're talking about vampires, you know? But this is regular blood, not the "ouch" kind. It's important to know that you are not dying, you're not injured, and you haven't hurt yourself. Getting your period is your body's way of saying everything is right on time and doing everything it's supposed to be doing.

And, let's just say, it can be super scary when you see that blood in your underwear the first time. For me, it was kind of scary. I mean, I knew my period was coming, but when I saw that blood—my mind just blanked out. I got a little woozy. I started seeing stars. I had to sit down right there on the tile floor. There was nothing in my brain—blank, zilch, nada, nothing—all I could think was, "I'm bleeding! I'm injured! Am I going to die? Is this how it all ends?" As you can see, I sort of, low-key panicked a little. But then finally, my mind relaxed a bit, and then I was like, "Oh wait, is that my period?..." And then, something magical happened! I got kind of excited, and then nervous, and then kind of excited again! A whole mixture of emotions washed over me. I'm telling you all of this because it's important for you to know that everybody has a different reaction, and whatever you feel is the right thing for you to feel. Just let your mind relax... and then think, "Wow, I'm growing up!"

But here's the exciting part: You'll get some pretty awesome perks and new skills as you grow from a cool kid into an even cooler adult.

Unlock Your Period Power!

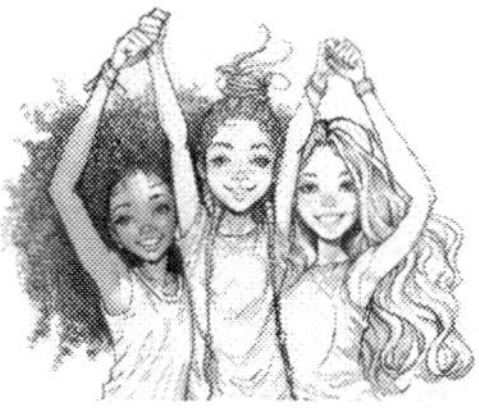

Super Strength: With each monthly wave of your period hormones (especially estrogen), these new chemicals rush through your body to make you become more muscular and your bones stronger. This upgrading of strength can only come with having the hormones that come with your period. Interesting, right?

Now, think back to those soccer skills we were just talking about—because of your period hormones, with practice, you can become stronger on the field. Because of these hormones, your body will develop more strength to show off its new superpowers! You're already mentally strong, but by getting physically stronger, you can tackle this thing and anything else life throws at you.

New Opportunities: Growing up means you might get to have more responsibility. When you show the ability to handle your period and take care of your body, your parents will probably recognize that you are ready to slowly make more of your own decisions and take on new privileges. Game on!

Emily's Epic Journey

Emily was just like you. When she got her period at 12 years old, she was not ready to swap out her kid card for the grown-up badge. She wanted to lock herself in her room and not leave until she could be a "kid" again. But after some heart-to-heart talks with her mom and big sister, she started seeing things differently. They shared their own stories with her, making her feel like she was part of something bigger, like a family tradition.

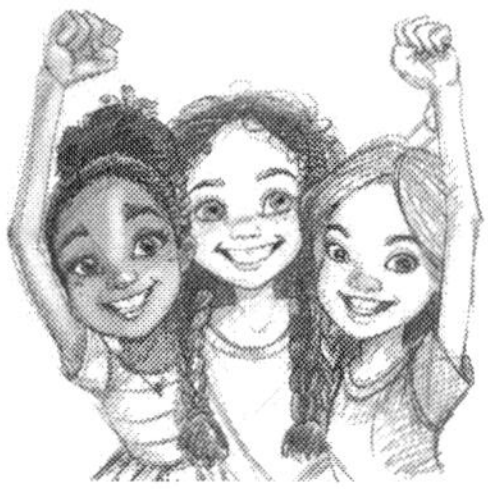

Emily got more into sports as she learned more about what her body could do and bonded with her body in a seriously cool way. She ran track for her school team, and her track stats got faster, and her body got stronger. She realized that growing up didn't mean ditching her kid self. It just meant adding more layers to who she already was.

Emily strutted home from school, all smiles after nailing a race. She realized that without her new upgraded body—yup, the one that dealt with periods and everything else—she wouldn't have been able to fly like the wind when it became "game-time." That day, she felt a kind of amazement about growing up. And, low-key, it felt like her body was nearing genius mode.

Your Exciting Future Awaits!

As you level up, you'll realize that each step is filled with opportunities to face new challenges, experiment with new things, and uncover your true strength. It's not about leaving kid-land behind. It's about growing into someone even more amazing. Sure, the road might look a little scary right now, but think of all the great adventures waiting for you. I mean, without your period, you can never become a mother. I know that's not on your schedule right now, but it's something pretty special to think about for the future.

With each step, you're not losing anything. Instead, you're stacking up more power, wisdom, and experience. Starting your period is only one chapter of the fantastic story of life that you're living. It's not the whole story, just one of many of its thrilling chapters. Now, take another deep breath, and let's take the next step in your great adventure!

ACTION TAKEAWAYS:

- Nobody learns everything all at once.
- Your period hormones help your body grow stronger.
- Exciting new opportunities and responsibilities await you.
- There's a lot to look forward to!
- Got questions? Talk it out with your parents or a trusted adult.

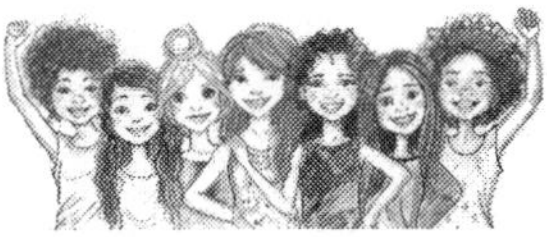

5. Period 101

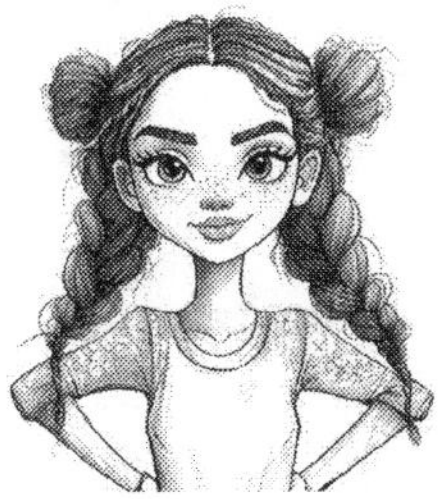

Welcome to the deep dive into all things period. We're talking about your monthly visitor, the ins, the outs, and the what-the-hecks moments of "that time of the month." We'll be talking more about those symptoms (because, let's face it, they are kind of crummy sometimes), choosing your period protection like a boss, and getting into the core of tracking your cycle. So, get ready because we're about to become Period Pros together!

The Menstrual Cycle: What's the Deal?

Your menstrual cycle is like the behind-the-scenes of a TikTok video. There's a lot is going on that you don't see. It's not only about the days you're actually menstruating. The big picture is that your whole menstrual cycle is built for a future baby-making scenario. It's got four main phases: Menstrual, Follicular, Ovulation, and Luteal phases. Sounds complicated, but it's pretty cool once you get the hang of it.

1. Menstrual Phase: This is the "main event" when you're *bleeding* during your period. It's your body's way of clearing the uterus lining because no baby happened this month. It's like someone yelled, "Party's over, y'all—everybody out!"

2. Follicular Phase: This phase starts on day one of your period and lasts until ovulation. Your body is prepping an egg within one of your ovaries to be the star of the show: The VIP.

3. Ovulation Phase: At the end of the follicular phase, your ovary releases the egg, called ovulation. This is the VIP guest (the egg) saying, "Ta-dah! Hello world, here I am!"

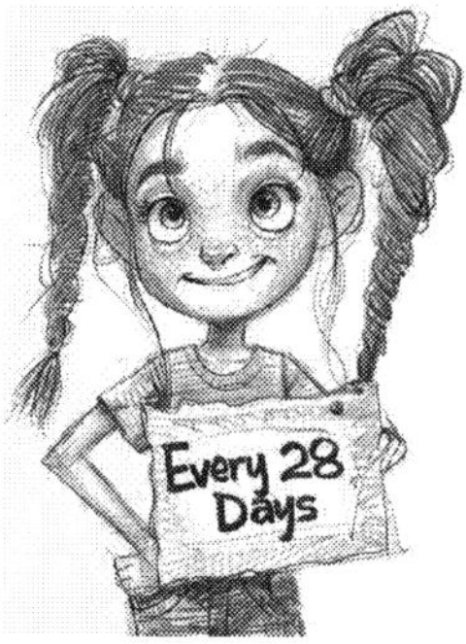

4. Luteal Phase: After the big debut above (ovulation), the luteal phase is where the VIP guest (the egg) leaves her home (the ovary), all dressed up in her party clothes, gets into the limo, and then makes her way through one of the fallopian tubes to get to where the party is happening (the uterus). This is where your body starts to prep for a baby or gets ready to start the cycle over again. If there's no baby, then your body says, "No problem!" Then the Menstrual Phase (#1 above) begins again and that guy screams, "Party's over, y'all—everybody out!" and the whole thing starts over with your period beginning again.

So, there it is! 1, 2, 3, 4, repeat! Easy-peasy!

Then, you'll want to put all that information in your ***MY PERIOD POWER! WORKBOOK.*** The workbook will explain how and where to put the information. Tracking your period symptoms is a large part of feeling comfortable with all this change.

Let's Get Some Facts

1. Usually, your period cycle lasts 28 days and is defined as the first day of your last period to the first day of your next period. But, the range can be from 21 to 35 days. This is still typical for someone in your age. And getting into a rhythm? It might take a while for your period to get on a regular schedule, but that's totally okay.
2. How long will my period last? Your period can last as few as three days and as many as eight days and still be normal. The average length of a period is five days. Not too shabby!
3. Do you think it's going to be a flood? No way! It might look like a lot, but it's only about three tablespoons throughout your whole period. That's about as much as three ketchup packets. Not as much as you thought, right?
4. All the eggs you'll ever have in your life are within your ovaries before you were even born! That's pretty incredible stuff!
5. Your period fluids only start to smell once they come in contact with the air. Super interesting, right?! Once the period blood gets exposed to oxygen, bacteria develops (Eww!). That's why we NEVER reuse any tampons, even if they only have little or no blood on them. Bacteria = Infection. (Aaaaargh!)
6. It's possible your period symptoms could get worse when the weather is cold.
7. Your voice and sense of smell can change a little during your period.
8. Will my period hurt? Even though you are bleeding, you are not injured. Any pain that you have would be mainly from cramping. Cramping is actually your uterus using its muscles to get rid of the unused lining because there was no baby. Cramping might hurt (sometimes) because your uterus doesn't use those muscles very often. It's like this: Say you went to

the gym and worked out your arms really, really hard. The next day, your arms are killing you! You can barely even lift a glass of water to your mouth. It's like that, but for your uterus.

9. The two main hormones we'll be talking about are estrogen and progesterone, and we'll chat about those more later.

Whew! I don't know about you, but these facts are incredibly interesting! The body is an amazing thing!

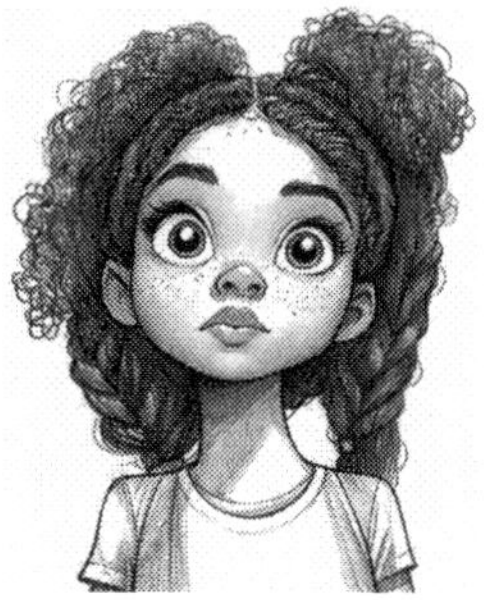

How Do I Know When My Period Is Coming?

Your body is so smart it will probably give you some hints that your period is coming. Who knew your body was such a genius? You might only get one of these hints or you might get a few of them, but it's cool to know that your body will give you an idea when it is coming. Preparation is important.

Here are some hints:

- **Eeeeeek, Acne!** The rising hormone levels in your body cause an extra amount of oil to be secreted, and it blocks some of the pores on your face. When you get extra pimples or blackheads, that's your "Alert! Alert! All hands on deck! Period is around the corner!"
- **Breasts Feeling a Little "Ouch?"** That's another big signal that your period is on the way.
- **Are You Feeling Tired but Finding it Hard to Sleep?** That's another signal that your period is coming soon. Fatigue (tiredness) is another part of having your period because your core temperature rises, especially when you're sleeping. It makes it difficult to get a good night's sleep. Your sleep

quality will improve after your period ends and your body temperature equalizes.

- **A Little Cramping** before your period starts is not uncommon, and can be a hint that your period is coming. Take this as a signal to stock up on your period supplies.
- **Discharge?** Before you start your period, you might see a clear-ish discharge on your underwear. That's a hint that your period is on its way.
- **Are You Constipated or Bloated?** Or do you have diarrhea or have gas? (Ugh, poop hints!) They might not happen, but they could.
- **Headaches?** Yep, it could be your period coming. Changes with that hormone that I mentioned earlier (estrogen) are another sign. Drinking a lot of water will help!
- **Mood Swings, Angry or Irritable?** Yup, can be another hint.
- **Feeling a Little Anxious or Depressed** can also be a hint that your period is coming.
- **Lower Back or Thigh Pain?** Sometimes, when you have cramps, it doesn't just hurt in your belly, but also in your lower back and even your thighs.

<u>IMPORTANT</u>: These are *POSSIBLE* hints. Don't freak out!!! You'll probably only get one or two of these, if that.

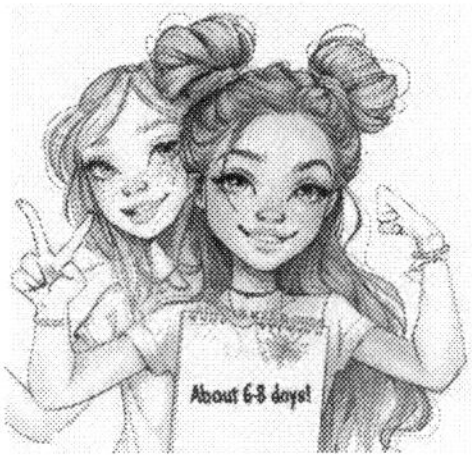

Choosing Your Period Protection: The Ultimate Showdown

We've already introduced the major players: Pads, tampons, and menstrual cups. We're going to talk more in-depth about how to use each of these in a later chapter, but let's get into some of the basic details, shall we?

- **Pads:** They come in different sizes and absorbencies. There are even ones designed for nighttime so you can sleep without worrying about leaks. You will learn more in the Pads chapter.
- **Tampons:** They also come in different absorbencies. The key is to change them regularly, every 4 to 6 hours, to avoid any health risks. If you're worried about forgetting, setting a timer on your phone can be a lifesaver. Literally. You should NEVER leave them inside for more than 6 hours. You will learn more about this in the tampons chapter.
- **Menstrual Cups:** They might seem advanced at first, but once you master inserting and removing them, you can wear them for up to 12 hours. They're eco-friendly since you're not throwing away pads or tampons. It might take a bit of practice, but there are tons of tutorials online can help. And of course, there is an upcoming menstrual cup chapter.

It's All About Absorbency

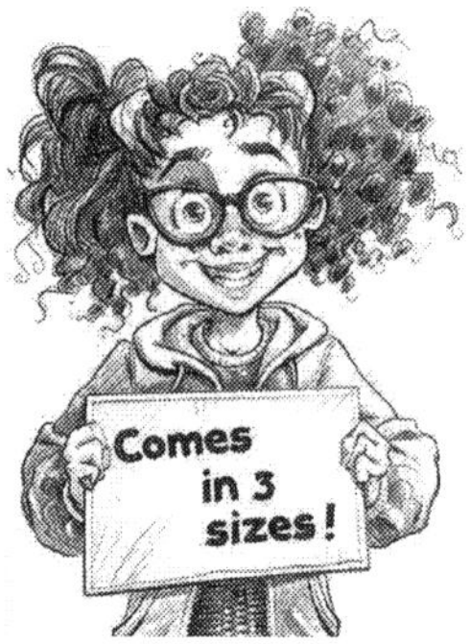

One last thing about period products: Picking the right absorbency is super important. Using something that's too absorbent can be uncomfortable and unnecessary. On the flip side, using something not absorbent enough can lead to leaks, which is pretty much the last thing you want. Here's the deal:

- **Light Absorbency:** This is perfect for those days when your flow is just saying "hello" or "goodbye." It is great for the start or end of your period when things are winding down.
- **Regular Absorbency:** This is your middle-of-the-road buddy. Most days, this will be your go-to. It's perfect for the average flow day and can handle your period without making you feel like you're wearing a diaper or risking a leak.
- **Super Absorbency:** For when it feels like your body is trying to make up for lost time. If you have heavy flow days (and

many of us do, it's very common), super absorbency products come to the rescue. Just remember, especially with tampons, to change them every 4-6 hours **(6 hours max)** to prevent health issues.

Wrap Up: Period Pro In Training

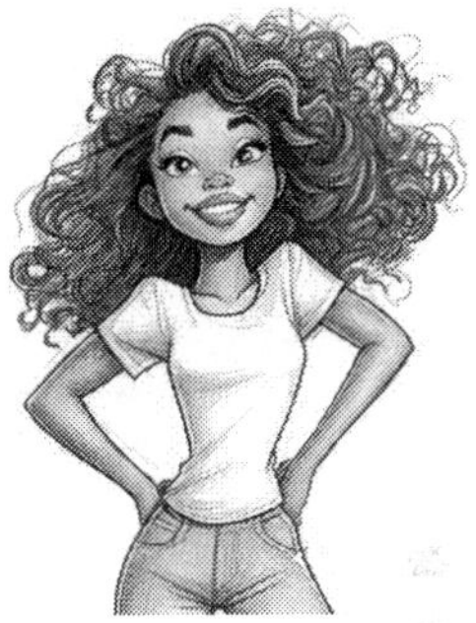

By now, you should be starting to understand some of this period stuff. Being armed with the "411" on your menstrual cycle should give you a warm feeling of confidence.

Everyone's experience with their period is different. What works for one person might not work for another. It's important to listen to your body, prepare yourself, and be open to trying different things until you find what makes your period a little more comfortable.

ACTION TAKEAWAYS:

- A period cycle is about 28 days from the first day of your period to the first day of your next period.
- When you're on your period, you are not injured or hurt.
- Your body will give you hints your period is coming.
- Keep checking out the various pads, tampons, menstrual cups.
- Pads and tampons come in light, regular, and super.
- You can track your period symptoms in the ***MY PERIOD POWER! WORKBOOK.***
- Talk about all these things to your Mom or a trusted adult to get the answers that you need.

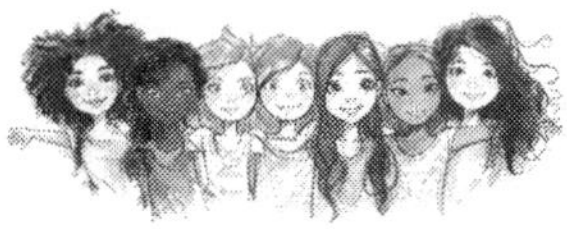

This Is Your Body!

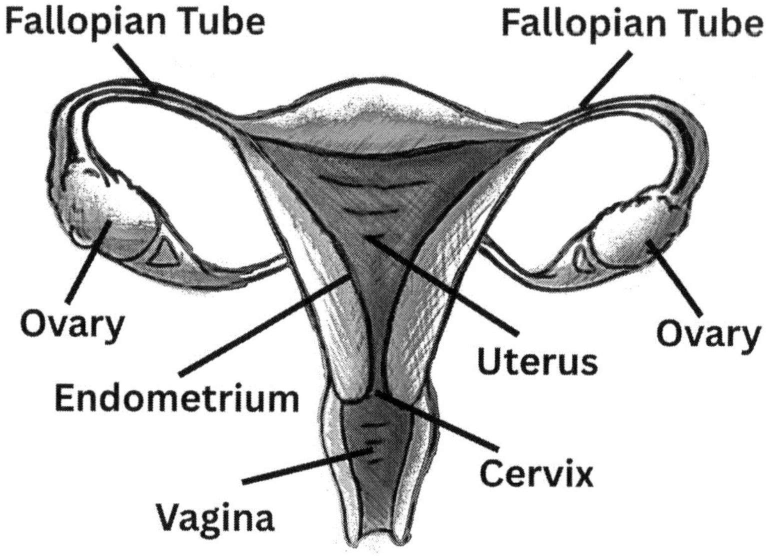

6. Pads -- How to Use the Period Products

PADS

When it's "that time of the month," you've got to be ready with your gear, right? Always make sure you have a stash of pads and pantyliners ready because you never know when it's going to sneak up on you. It's like preparing for a surprise test!

What Are Pads Made Of?

Pads consist mainly of layers of absorbent materials. The main part is usually made of cotton, which is soft and comfy. Then, there's a super absorbent polymer layer inside. It soaks up all the fluids like magic! Most of them have a plastic backing to prevent leaks. There's usually an adhesive strip on that plastic backing so you can attach it to your underwear.

Pantyliners

Okay, so I know we haven't really talked about these things, but they are super useful. Pantyliners are like the scouts of the period world—

always prepared! These little guys are always on the front lines when things are just starting out or almost done. They are super thin and kind of feel like nothing, which is cool. You simply peel off the paper backing (it makes a satisfying zip sound), and stick it in your underwear. Make sure it's smack dab in the middle to catch everything. It's kind of like placing a sticker in your favorite notebook, but you know, not.

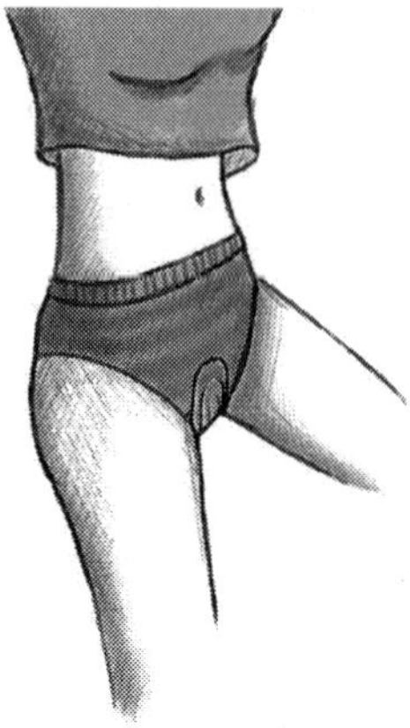

Pads

These are the real MVPs when things get, um, heavier. They're also the things that you will probably use almost all the time when you first start out because they are super easy to use. They come in different sizes, anything from ultra-thin to overnight pads. Go to the store and study them a bit, and choose the ones you'll need. You might try out different sizes and brands until you find the ones you like. They are all a little different from each other. Then, from your stash, you see how your day is going and decide which absorbency to use—like choosing armor for battle.

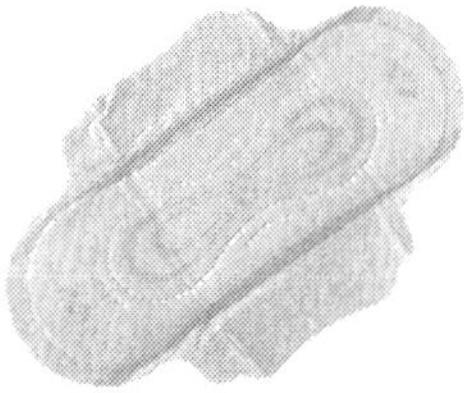

The bigger pads are for the heavy days, and the smaller ones are for when it's just chilling out. Same deal with these: You peel off the strip of paper and stick them to your underwear. Sometimes, there are wings on the sides of pads. Wings are these extra side-flaps that fold over the sides of your underwear to keep the pad in place to protect your undies. The wings give your underwear a "little hug" to make sure the pad doesn't go on a journey.

Reusable Pads—The Superhero Around the World!

Reusable pads are a total game-changer for people all over the globe, especially where it's like a treasure hunt to find period products. Imagine not being able to find a pad or tampon whenever you need one. Tough, right? That's where reusable pads swoop in and save the day.

Reusable pads are like the eco-friendly heroes of period products. Just like your favorite jacket, they have snaps that fasten around your underwear, so they stay put, no matter if you're killing it at sports or chilling with friends.

How do you keep these pads clean and ready for action? After using one, rinse it in cold water to wash it out. Then, you can toss it in the washing machine with your regular laundry. Super simple, right? Just skip the fabric softener and bleach because they stop absorption. Sunlight is a great way to dry them—it helps get rid of stubborn stains, helps keep the bacteria away, and keeps them fresh.

How many should you have? Well, it depends on your flow and how often you want to do laundry. Usually, having around 8 to 12 pads is a great start. This way, you've got enough to last your entire period without having to wash them every day.

Reusable pads are not only about saving the planet; they're about giving you the freedom to do your thing without the stress of having to find disposable pads all the time. Reusable pads are pretty much the superheroes of the period world!

Disposing of Pads and Pantyliners

This is important! NEVER flush them down the toilet. It will jam up your plumbing system, and your parents might kill you! After you're done, roll it up like a little burrito in its original wrapper or toilet paper. Never throw it in the trash can without this burrito move. This is also to be kind to others who might accidentally look into the trash can after

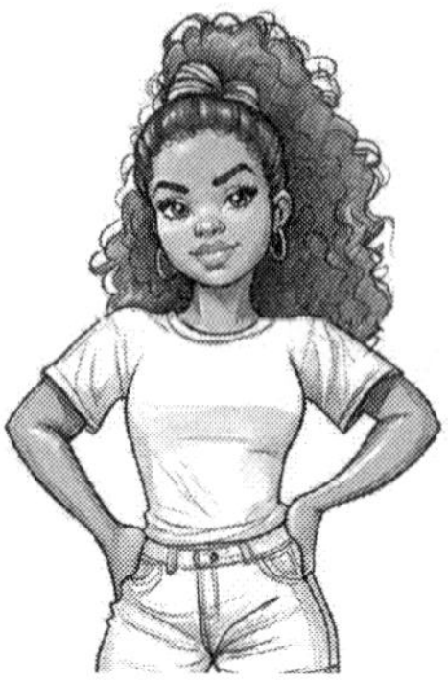

you have left the bathroom. Most bathrooms outside your home have a special bin for this stuff, so use it. It's like a secret disposal unit for girls, but you know, not so secret (haha!) And remember, wash your hands.

That's pretty much it for pads. Super easy, right? That's why people love them. They're really simple to use! You replace your gear every few hours, and you've nailed it. It's kind of like a rite of passage, getting to know all this stuff. Welcome to the club!

BONUS PRO TIP:
Wearing tight fitting underwear with pads can help keep them in place, or buy period panties.

ACTION TAKEAWAYS:

- Go shopping for pads and pantyliners. Compare the brands, sizes and styles until you find ones you like.
- Purchase a zippered, non-see-through pouch to store your away-from-home period products in. This is if it falls out of your backpack, no one will see what's inside. So embarrassing!
- Don't reuse any period products, even if they look only slightly used.
- Use the burrito move to dispose of your pads.
- **NEVER** flush them down the toilet!
- And remember, wash your hands!

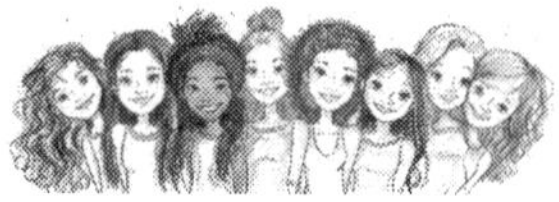

7. Tampons to the Rescue!

What Are Tampons?

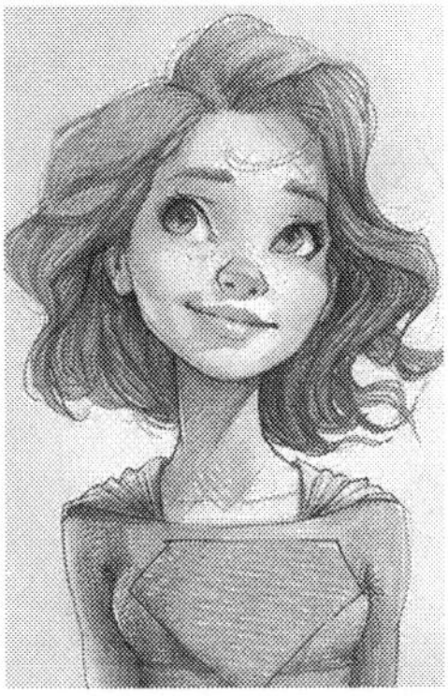

Tampons are little cotton tubes that you can use during your period to soak up the blood. They are small, and you put them inside your body. They come with a string at the end to help you take them out easily and are super handy if you want to swim or play sports, because they stay hidden and don't get in the way. Just remember to change them every few hours to stay fresh and comfy.

IMPORTANT:

Read this entire chapter (all eight sections) before you try your first tampon. Give yourself plenty of time. You don't want to rush it. This is "Big Step" time! You've got this!

What Are Tampons Made Of?

Manufacturers usually make tampons from cotton or a mix of cotton and rayon. They're made from some of the same stuff clothes are made from, which helps soak up the period blood really well.

They Come In These Sizes:

- **Junior/Slim/Slender:** These are good for when you're just starting to use a tampon. Because they are skinnier, they're easier to put inside. These are also good for when you're having a very light flow.
- **Regular:** These are for an average flow. You'll probably use these the most.
- **Super:** These are for when you have a heavy flow day. You're probably not going to need these very often.
- **Ultra/Super Plus:** These are for the rare days when you are having an extremely heavy flow. You will only want to use these once you're very experienced in using tampons. They are a bit large.

Tampons also come in two styles: With an applicator and without. The applicator is a handy tool to help you insert it without needing to put your fingers inside your body. But after a while, you'll get used to the idea, and you will decide which style of tampon you want to use.

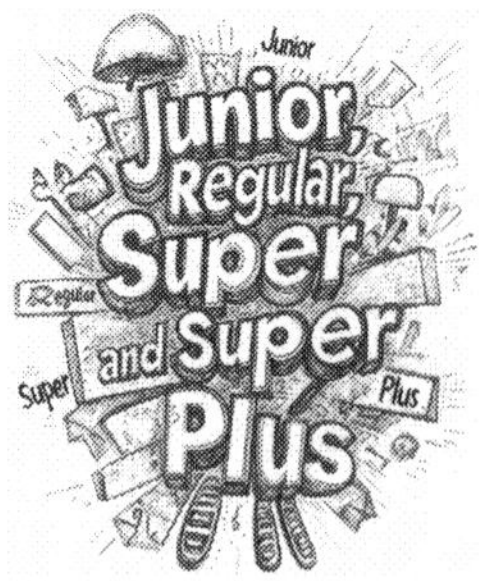

Why Use Tampons?

Sometimes, tampons are cool because you can swim with them and they are less bulky than pads. You don't really feel them once they are inside. Kind of amazing, right? Not feeling them? Yeah, it's true!

Lots of people wait to use tampons until they feel ready or are older. It's totally a personal choice. Sometimes, it takes a bit of time to get cozy with the idea of using tampons, no lie. It took me a while. So, no pressure.

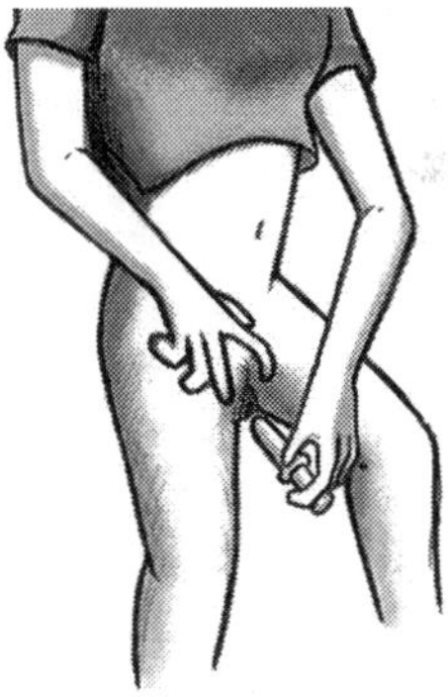

Let's Do This!

Step 1. Wash your hands!

Step 2. Different Ways to Stand While Inserting

1. The Flamingo: You can try standing with one foot on the toilet seat.
2. Mini Squat: Squatting down a little (slightly bending your knees apart) with both feet on the floor.
3. The Throne Sit: You can sit on the toilet with your knees apart and put your hands down within the bowl of the toilet. Don't touch the water with your hand or your tampon.

Step 3. The Angle

Imagine there's a line from the entrance of your vagina aiming towards the small of your back. That's the direction that you want to go. NOT STRAIGHT UP, but more like aiming towards your lower back.

Step 4A. How To Insert a Tampon WITH an Applicator

1. Find your "Zen" zone. Chill out and find a comfy spot in the bathroom. Breathe in… breathe out… take it slow. If you're feeling rushed, don't do it. Save it for later and wear a pad. But, if you have the time to take it slow and easy, then proceed to the next step.
2. Take the tampon out of its wrapper.
3. You will see the applicator, which is a plastic or a cardboard tube that helps the tampon slide in easier.
4. Hold the applicator with your thumb and middle finger near the grip (the middle part of the applicator, which sometimes has little lines or dots to help you hold it better).
5. Use your other hand and gently spread open the skin around your vagina.
6. Gently slide the tampon inside you. It might take a little bit of time the first couple of times. That's okay, take as long as you need. Be patient with yourself. This is all new stuff you're doing here, and it might feel kind of weird.
7. Once you have the tampon inserted correctly inside you, while you're gripping the outer tube, slowly push the inner tube up with your pointer finger or your other hand, sliding it into the outer tube until it comes to sort of a stop. Pause… take a breath… and think to yourself, "I did it!"
8. Once it's all the way in, pull out both tubes (the inner tube should automatically come out along with the outer tube).
9. SIDE TIP: Once you have completely inserted the tampon and have removed the tubes, you should actually feel nothing. The only feeling you might have is the slight amount of feeling from the string as it exits your body. If you feel something on the inside of your body, or if you experience any pain or discomfort, then you haven't inserted it correctly. If so, then dang, you'll need to remove it and start again with a new tampon. Same as before, check below for instructions on how to dispose of your used tampons.

Step 4B. How To Insert a Tampon WITHOUT an Applicator

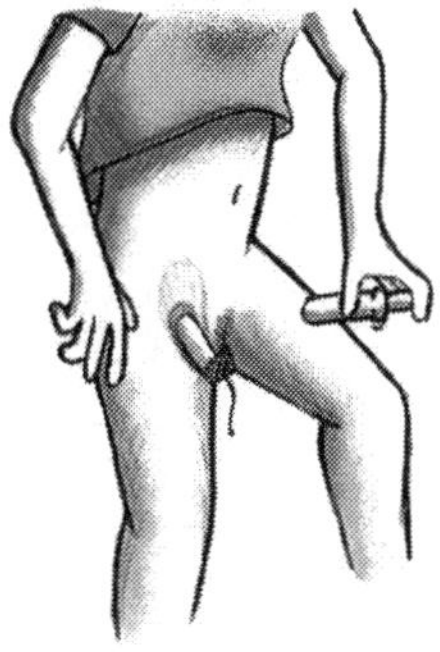

1. Once again, wash your hands. It's like the golden rule!
2. Find a relaxing spot where you feel totally at ease, like your bathroom at home.
3. Unwrap your tampon. You'll notice there's no applicator this time. It's just you and the tampon getting ready to team up.
4. Hold the tampon with your thumb and middle finger at the base (the end where the string comes out).
5. Use your other hand to hold the skin around your vagina open. It's prep time for the mission ahead.
6. As before, gently slide the tampon inside you, using your middle finger to guide it. Make sure it's sitting pretty far up there. (Yes, your finger will need to be inside you.) It might take a little bit of time the first couple of times. That's okay. Be patient with yourself and take as long as you need.
7. <u>SAME SIDE TIP</u>: Once you fully insert the tampon and remove your finger, you shouldn't feel anything. You might notice the string as it hangs outside your body. However, if you feel any discomfort or anything unusual inside you, it means you didn't insert the tampon properly. In that case, you'll have to remove it and try inserting a different one again. Check below for instructions on how to dispose of your used tampons.
8. You've got this! It's really the same steps, just without the applicator!

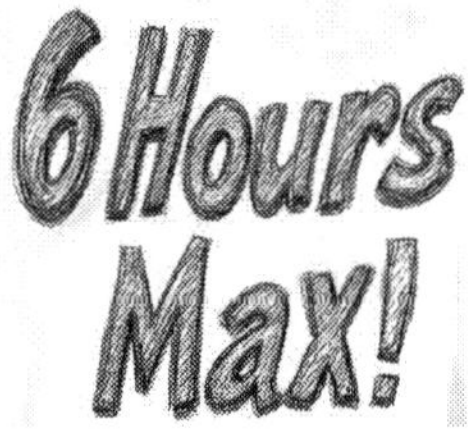

Step 5. How Long Can It Be Left In?

Keep your tampon in for **6 hours MAX.** This is a hard and set rule—NO MORE THAN 6 HOURS! 4 hours is better. You can set a timer on your phone to remind you to change your tampon, if you like. It will keep your body fresh and healthy. Changing it regularly is key to your success. I know you're going to do this right, rockstar!

Step 6. How to Take the Tampon Out

Okay, compadre, it's go time!

- Take a deep breath and relax your body like a quickie meditation.
- Gently pull on the string at a steady pace. It should slide out smoothly… Mission accomplished!

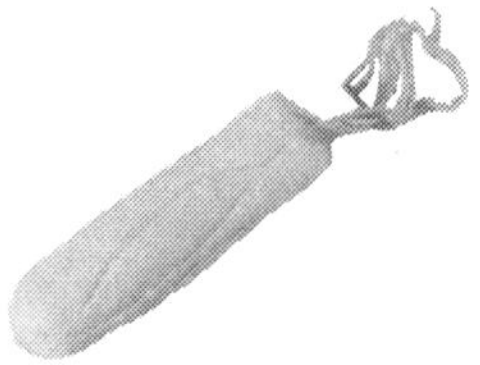

Step 7. How to Dispose of a Tampon

Wrap it up in toilet paper like a little burrito, just like how you did your pads. Use enough toilet paper and then give it a secret send-off into the garbage can, same as pads. These little guys should NEVER BE FLUSHED down the toilet! They can cause a plumbing disaster, and no one wants to call in a plumber, especially for a tampon rescue mission. How embarrassing that would be when the plumber pulls out a tampon! Yikes! Your parents would kill you—again!

Then, guess what? Ready for the next tampon? The whole thing happens again! It's always good to have your next tampon ready and waiting outside of the package so you can have easy and convenient insertion. Cool! You're really making things happen here!

Step 8. Wash your hands!

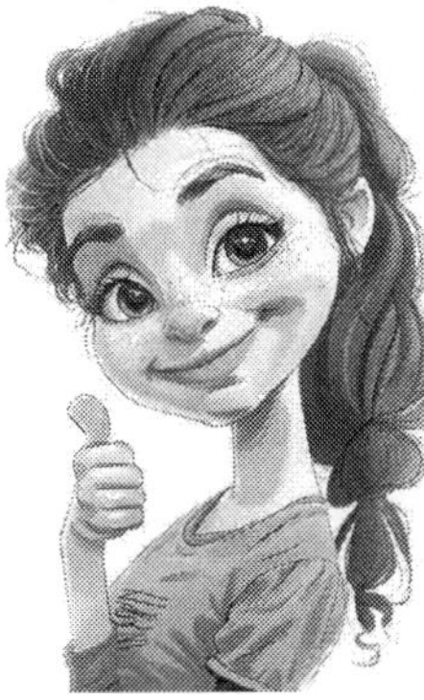

Wow! You Did It!

I have to tell you, navigating the world of tampons, especially non-applicator tampons, is a skill. The non-applicator tampons are really nice because they're small and easy to hide in your backpack. But you have to be okay with the whole "finger inside you" part. Tampons might feel tricky at first, but with a bit of practice, you'll find they become just another part of your period power tool kit. You're in the driver's seat. Go at your own pace and go with the products that feel right for you.

ACTION TAKEAWAYS:

- Read this entire chapter (all eight sections) before you try your first tampon.
- Go shopping for tampons. Compare the brands, sizes, and styles until you find ones that you like.
- Purchase a zippered, non-see-through pouch to store your away-from-home period products in. This is in case it falls out of your backpack, no one will see what's inside. Total blush moment!
- Don't reuse any period products, even if they only have a little blood on them.
- Only wear them for 4 to 6 hours. No more than 6 hours (MAX). 4 hours is better!
- Set a timer on your phone to remind you to change your tampons if you need to.
- NEVER flush them down the toilet!
- Wash your hands!
- Get help from a trusted adult—your Mom, sister, or someone

else who knows the ropes to learn the proper angle for tampon insertion.

- There's a lot going on with this period stuff, so ask questions!

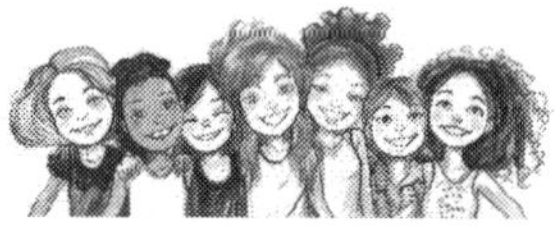

8. The Mysterious Menstrual Cup

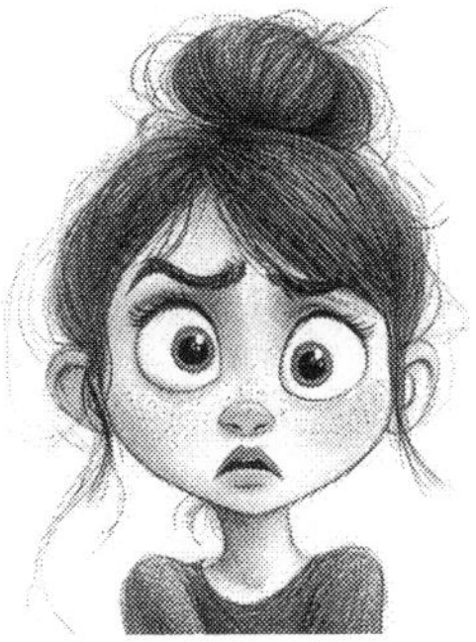

Hey superstars! Are you ready to investigate the eco-friendly world of menstrual cups? Think of them as the ninja warriors of period protection—sleek, smart, and super stealthy. Let's unravel the mystery and discover why these little guys are a worldwide lifesaver for menstruation.

But first, I'm not going to lie, menstrual cups are pretty advanced for someone just starting out. They can be a little intimidating even for someone who has been on their period for years. At this point, you're just starting to get used to the idea of blood coming out every month. Am I right? So, let's tiptoe into the world of menstrual cups and see if they are right for us.

What Exactly is a Menstrual Cup?

Imagine a tiny, flexible cup shaped like a bell. They're made of silicone or rubber, and this little hero sits snugly inside you, waiting to catch your flow. No mess, no waste, nothing to wrap up in toilet paper.

Once it's in, it's just total comfort. All you have to do is wash and reuse. You're not only saving the planet one pad at a time, but also saving money without having to purchase all the other products over and over. And, menstrual cups can last for years, if properly cared for.

IMPORTANT:

Read all seven steps in this chapter before trying to insert a menstrual cup for the first time. The menstrual cup takes some getting used to.

How to Become a Cup Pro

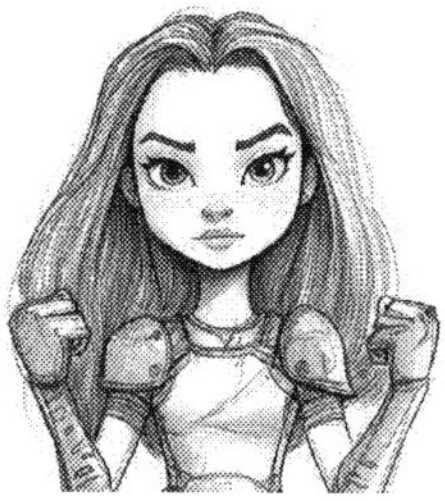

Becoming a menstrual cup pro might seem as tricky as learning to ride a bike for the first time, but with a bit of practice, you'll get it down. Here's how to master the menstrual cup from start to finish:

Step 1: Picking the Perfect Cup

First things first, choose a cup that fits your flow and your body. They come in different sizes, usually small and large, based on your age and flow intensity. When it's properly inserted, it will sit like an upside-down bell.

Step 2: Wash Your Hands

Step 3: Get in the Fold

To make insertion a breeze, you've got to fold it right. Here are the top two crowd-pleasers:

1. The U-Fold (or C-Fold): Fold the cup in half and press the sides of the cup together to form a "U" or "C" shape—easy peasy, lemon squeezy!

2. Push-Down Fold: Press down on the rim to the base to form a narrow point. This one is perfect for newbies since it makes the cup more slim!

IMPORTANT NOTE:

Even when folded, these little guys are wider than a tampon. You will not like using a menstrual cup until you are completely comfortable using a tampon. Menstrual cups are not for the newbie. Take your time. No rush.

Step 4: We're Going In!

Relax your muscles like you're about to float in a pool. Are you ready? If so, find a comfy squat or put one foot up on the toilet seat, and gently guide the cup in, rim first. Push it gently toward your lower back, using your finger to guide it. Make sure it pops open to create a leak-proof seal. (You must check it inside you with your finger to see if it is a good seal.) Get more information online to get specific instructions, pictures, and videos about menstrual cup folding. Then—Voilà! It's in!

Step 5: Wash Your Hands

INSIGHT: Do I Have It In Right?

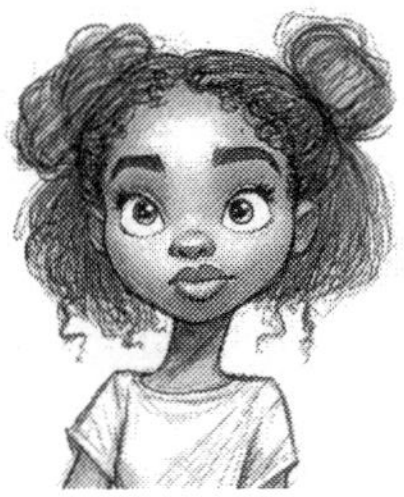

To know if you have it in right, you should basically feel nothing. The only thing you might feel is the little tail at the bottom of the cup, but that's about it. If you feel something inside you, then you probably don't have it in right, and you will need to remove it and try it once again.

It's important that it fits snugly inside you and feels like a slight suction against where your flow comes out. Testing it means that you'll have to put your finger(s) inside you. You, being a new period pro, might not be okay with all this "finger inside you stuff" and that's okay. Like I said in the beginning of this chapter, this is really an advanced technique.

Step 6: Live Your Life

Once inside, menstrual cups can stay in place for up to 12 hours, but I really recommend it to be closer to 8-10 hours. That means that you can wear it overnight. With these little guys, you can dance, swim, run, and even sleep without worry. Your cup has your back!

Step 7: Removal

Need to remove it? Stay calm and carry on! Pinch the base to release the seal. (It's important to release the seal, because it creates a bit of suction in there.) To pinch the base, your finger(s) will probably need to be inside you. Ignore the stem. That's only for finding it. Wiggle it gently and pull it out. Empty into the toilet, give it a good rinse, and either pop it back in or give it a good wash for next time.

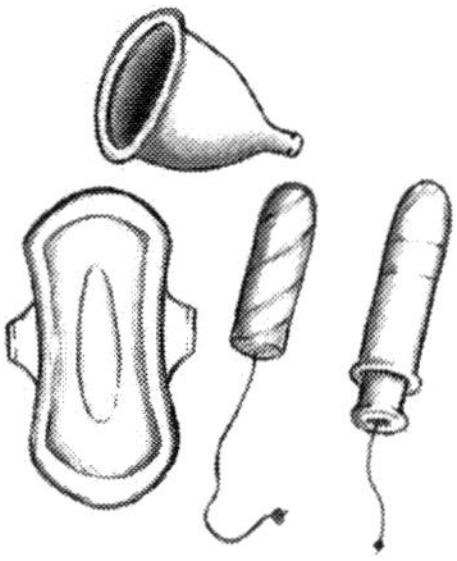

Cup Cleaning Tips

- **Regular Rinses:** Wash your cup with mild soap and water each time you empty it.
- **End-of-Cycle:** Boil your cup for 5-10 minutes at the end of your period to keep it germ-free and ready for next time. Read your menstrual cup manufacturer's directions on how to take care of it.
- **Storage:** To keep your cup happy and healthy, store it in a breathable fabric pouch. Avoid airtight containers.

Cup Traveling Tips:

- **Back-Up Buddy:** Having an extra cup means always being prepared. You can rotate them to make sure they are germ-free.
- **Travel Tactics:** Pack a small bottle of water to rinse your cup in public restrooms. Keep your cup pouch handy for quick stashes.

Navigating the world with your menstrual cup is more than period protection. It's about empowerment, eco-friendliness, and embracing your body's capabilities. So, gear up with your favorite cup (if you're ready for this step) and celebrate your amazing self!

Wrapping It All Up on Period Products

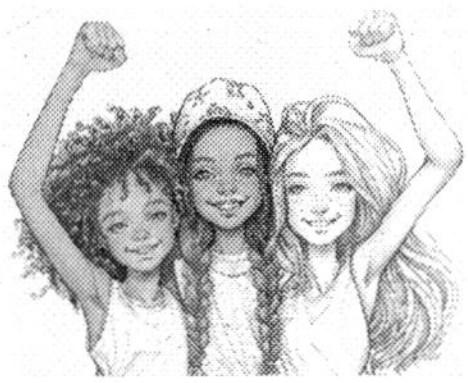

Okay, Sunshine! Whew! That was a lot of information! There's a lot of physical stuff to get used to, I know. Just take it slow and easy. No rush to get into tampons or even menstrual cups. Whether you use pads, tampons, menstrual cups, or a combination of the three, when you're ready, you can rock your period like the queen you are. Go at your own pace. Let your confidence shine as bright as your sparkling personality! Everything is based on your decision timeline. You've got this!

ACTION TAKEAWAYS:

- Read all seven steps in this chapter before trying to insert a menstrual cup for the first time.
- Read the instructions and try it out if you're ready.
- There is no rush to try menstrual cups. Go at your own pace.
- Get more information online to get specific instructions, pictures, and videos about menstrual cup folding.

- Order different sizes of period products ahead of time, and practice the folds before you try to use it.
- Get a fabric pouch with a zipper or a drawstring closure to keep your menstrual cup in.
- During your period, you can quickly rinse your cup, but at the end of your period, you should boil your cup in water using the manufacturer's instructions.
- Wash your hands!
- Using menstrual cups is pretty advanced. Please reach out to someone to get a personal demonstration on how to fold the cup, or look online and really study the videos.
- Please talk this stuff out with your mom, your sister, or your doctor. Get the answers you need!

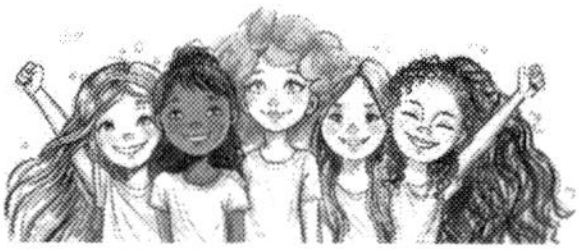

9. Let's Be Serious... Just For a Moment, I Promise

Okay team, it's time to get a tad serious and chat about something super important: Keeping yourself safe and sound during your period.

I know, I know, we've been on a fun ride with all the jokes and cool hacks, but this stuff? It's major league important. It's like the ultimate bad guy that you've got to be fully prepared for.

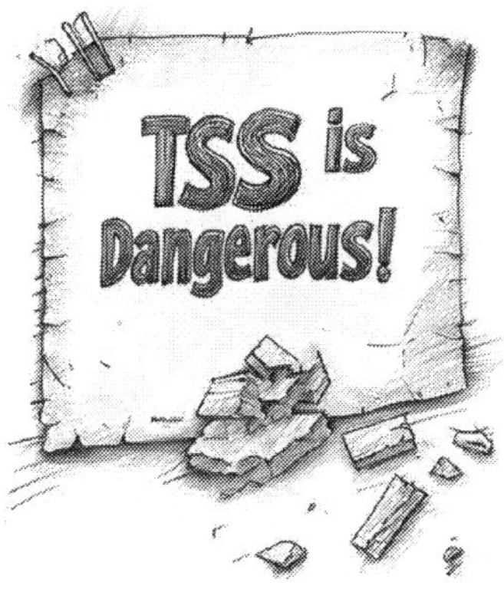

What's the Deal with Toxic Shock Syndrome (TSS)?

You've probably seen those warnings on tampon boxes and wondered, "What's the big deal?"

TSS (Toxic Shock Syndrome) is like the villain in superhero movies—**rare, but extremely serious.** This is a condition where bacteria (yuck!) go a bit wild and produce serious toxins in your body. It's not the party you want to be hosting.

TSS—The Lowdown

TSS happens when bacteria (the bad guys) produce toxins in your body, which can get very serious if it's not treated. One way to get TSS is by leaving a tampon in for too long. Yep, that's why all those tampon boxes say, **"change every 4 to 6 hours."**

Pro Tips to Dodge TSS:

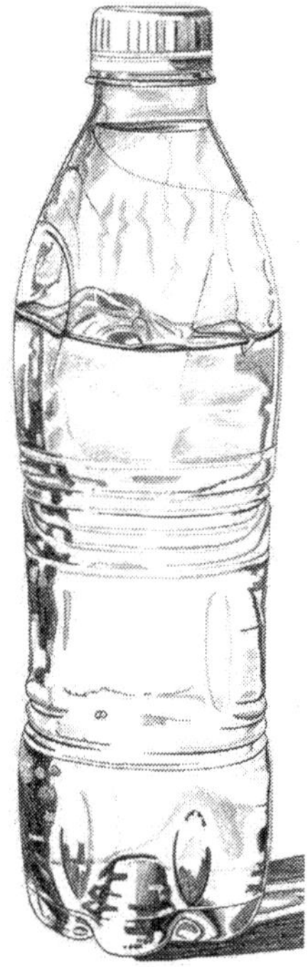

- **Water is Your Best Friend:** I know, I've said it before, and I know I'll probably say it again, but it's really important. Chug that H2O (water)! It's the secret potion that helps with bloating and can even make cramps and headaches take a hike. It keeps your fluids moving, which is what you need during your period.
- **Timely Tampon Changes:** Stick to changing your tampon every 4 to 6 hours, even on those light flow days. **Even if it feels like you could go longer, just don't.** It's like resetting your video game timer to avoid "Game Over."
- **Pick the Right Absorbency:** Using a tampon that is too absorbent for your flow will up your risk. It's important to get the correct size tampon for your flow. Using a super absorbent tampon on a light day is like wearing a snowsuit in the summer. It's uncomfy and unnecessary. This is definitely not a time to think big.
- **Don't Reuse:** This may sound obvious to some of us, but it's important to say. If you pull out a tampon and there's barely any blood on it, it's important not to reuse it. This is not a time to save money. Once the tampon leaves your body, it immediately begins creating bacteria.

- **Mix It Up:** Consider rotating between pads and tampons. Your body will thank you for the variety.

BONUS PRO TIP:

Set a timer on your phone if you think you might forget to change your tampon. The timer goes off, and you change your tampon. After that, you can reset the timer again. You're golden!

Choosing Your Period Gear Wisely

With a bazillion period products out there, finding your perfect match is key. But, like any good relationship, communication (with your body), keeping safe is very important.

- **Read the Instructions!** Give those product instructions a good read. It might not be as fun as scrolling TikTok, but it's essential to know how to use each of them safely.
- **Listen to Your Body:** If a product makes you feel itchy, uncomfortable, or just plain wrong, your body is trying to send you an SOS signal—"Help Me!" Your body is like your BFF—if it's trying to tell you something, listen up, chica!

If you need to talk to a grown-up or a doctor, please do it. They're your support team. They're there to help you build your game plan.

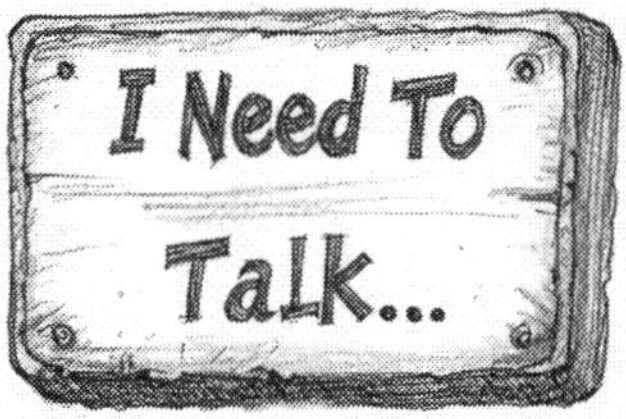

You're a Woman Now

Yup, you heard that right! (Eeeeek!) Your body is doing womanly things, and beginning your period also means that IF you become sexually active (which means sexual intercourse) with a member of the opposite sex, you could get pregnant.

IMPORTANT: Let's state that again because it's really important—**you could get pregnant**.

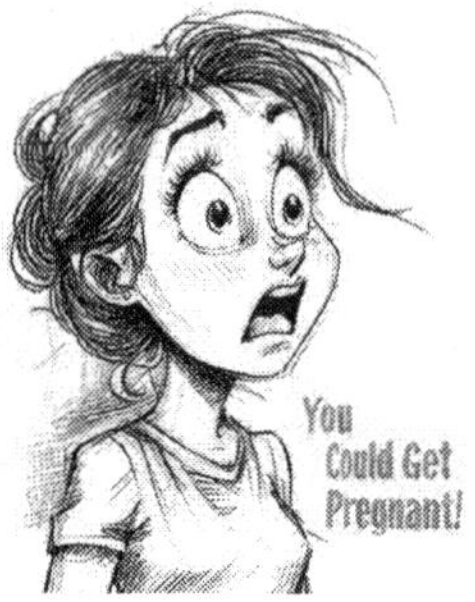

Now, considering that this is a book about getting your first period, getting to know how your body functions, and everything that goes along with this beautiful transition into adulthood, having intercourse and getting pregnant is probably not on your immediate list of things to do. However, you need to be aware that the possibility of pregnancy is a real situation if you are sexually active.

We're not really going to cover sex or pregnancy topics in detail in this book because that's a very large subject with a lot of personal (and even religious) decisions you need to make. However, it is something that you need to know. When the time is right later in your development, you will want to talk about it with your parents and your doctor BEFORE becoming sexually active.

It is never too soon to have real conversations like these with the people you trust to give you good advice and guidance.

The Final Boss: Your Health

Okay, deep breath in, and hold it… hold it… and let it out! Go ahead, I'll wait… Aaaaaaaah, feels good, right? These are some tough subjects, but calm breathing helps you find your Zen again.

See, peeps? We made it through the serious stuff! It wasn't so scary, was it? Knowing how to keep yourself safe during your period is like unlocking the final level in a game of Period Land.

Taking care of your health during your period isn't just about battling the bad guys like TSS, or dealing with cramps; it's also about listening to your body, making smart choices, staying clean, keeping an eye on your time, setting alarms, and knowing when to ask for help. It's about

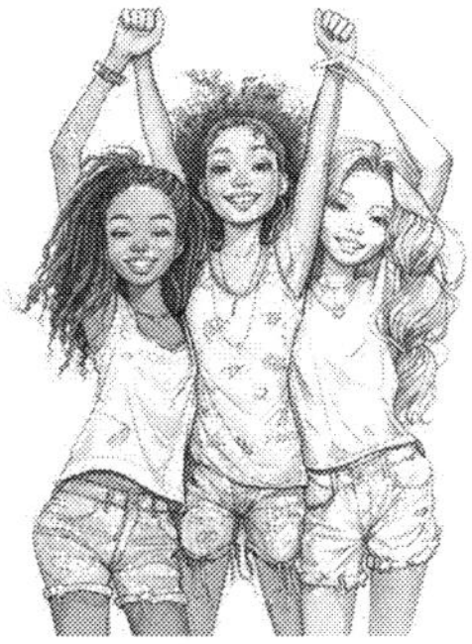

getting guidance before becoming sexually active. It means you get to be the hero in your own story.

So, keep on keeping on, you amazing, well-informed, health-savvy warrior! Your period is only one part of the incredible journey of being you. Stay safe and stay smart, and guess what? You're not only getting through your period—you're mastering it. High-fives all around! You've totally got this!

ACTION TAKEAWAYS:

- Change your tampon every 4 to 6 hours (MAX).
- Set timers on your phone to help you remember when to change your tampon.
- Never reuse period products, even if there's only a little blood on them.
- Wash your hands.
- Hydrate!
- Talk to your parents and doctor BEFORE becoming sexually active because you could get pregnant.
- Listen to your body. It's probably telling you something!

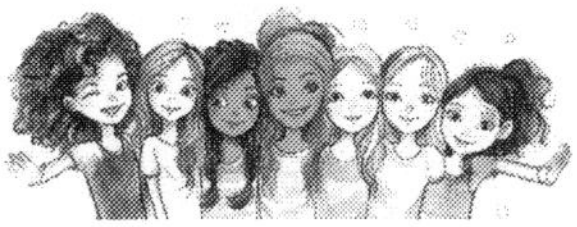

10. The Emotional Rollercoaster (Sometimes...)

Welcome to the chapter where we talk about what's even trickier than deciding whether to use a pad or a tampon: The Emotional Roller-coaster. Yeah, I'm talking about those times when you cry at a commercial or laugh hysterically at a spoon. Because it's hormones. Yeah.

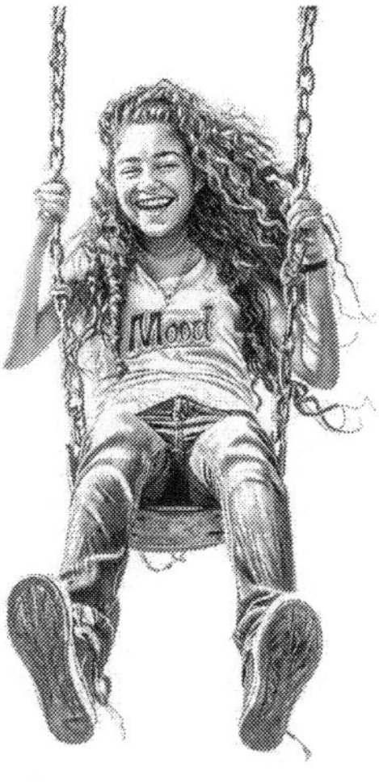

We're now going to go deeper into managing the emotional ups and downs that come with periods, get rid of more myths, and give you more tips on building that all-important support system.

Hormones: The Invisible Puppet Masters

First, let's talk about why you're feeling all the feels. Hormones are like your body's text messages sending signals to different parts of your body during your menstrual cycle. During your menstrual cycle, these hormone levels go up and down, basically throwing a party in your body without asking permission. *Rude much?*—yeah, I know. Anyway, this can make you feel super happy one minute and then totally down the next. It's not you, it's your hormones. Understanding this will help you prepare for the mood swings.

These hormones are called estrogen and progesterone, and they are natural chemicals your body creates to tell it what to do. These are the chemicals that actually start your puberty rolling, which is your body waking up to becoming an adult. All of this is happening while your brain is screaming, "I'm not ready yet!" Don't worry, it's a gradual process.

We're going to talk more about these hormones later, but the important part to understand here is that those hormones going up and down inside you each month are what are yanking your mood all around. Sometimes making you silly, sometimes angry, and sometimes sad.

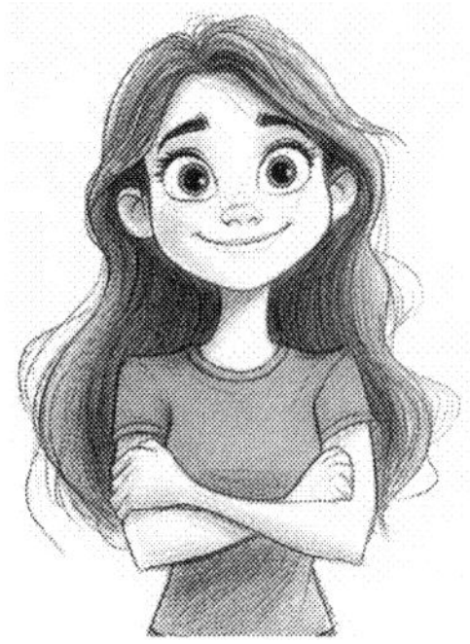

- **What's Happening Inside:** Right before your period, your estrogen and progesterone levels drop, which can make you feel you're in an emotional tidal wave. They can make you feel more emotional or sensitive. It's like your body's way of saying, "Heads up, things are about to get real!"
- **Listen to Your Body and Your Mind (Period Tracking):** These emotional roller coaster hints are important information that you will want to document in your Mood Diary within the ***MY PERIOD POWER! WORKBOOK.*** This info will help you figure out your needs for later months. It will help you get a handle on how to give your body some love during difficult times. Just like you track your period and track your moods, after a few months, you might see a pattern. For example: Say you notice that the third day of every period is a bit difficult emotionally—write it down! Tracking that third day will help

you plan for when you might need a little extra self-care or know when to carry extra snacks.

- **Dealing with Mood Swings:** Sharing your feelings with friends or family can be super helpful. It's okay to feel all over the place.
- **Create a Coping Toolbox:** Have a list of things that make you feel better for those tough days. It could be a playlist of your favorite music, a cozy blanket, or a list of funny videos that always make you laugh.
- **Write it Down:** Sometimes you feel you can't talk to anyone, that you don't know if you can trust them. You can also write all those feelings that are bubbling up within you in your ***MY PERIOD POWER! WORKBOOK.*** This workbook is where you can share all your feelings because you are talking to YOU. You are talking only to yourself. Plus, there are fun games, beautiful coloring pages, silly jokes, mazes, journaling, recipes, and girlfriend stuff! I got you!

Myth Busters: Period Edition

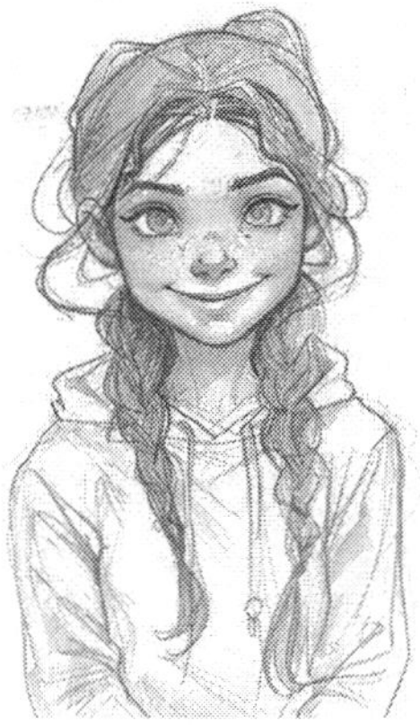

There's a lot of weird stuff people say about periods, and most of it's not true. Like, no, you can't hold a period in like pee (yes, someone people actually think that). And no, sharks won't attack you if you swim in the ocean during your period.

Busting Myths:

Let's get one thing straight—periods are normal, natural, and nothing to be ashamed of. Learning the facts can help you feel more confident when your periods come and can help you educate others.

- **Myth:** You can't swim when you're on your period. Totally false. With the right products, like tampons or menstrual cups, you can swim, dance, and do everything you usually do.
- **Myth:** Period blood is dirty. Nope, it's just blood and tissue your body doesn't need right now. There's nothing dirty or shameful about it.
- **Myth:** If you hang out with other girls, your periods will sync up. This is a weird one that doesn't have solid science backing it up. It's more coincidence than anything else.

There are other myths, of course. If you have questions, talk to your parents, your doctor, or research online.

Dealing With the Stigma:

If someone makes a weird comment about your period, remember, they are the ones being weird, not you. Own your body and your knowledge, and don't let myths or people make you feel embarrassed.

Supercharging Your Support System

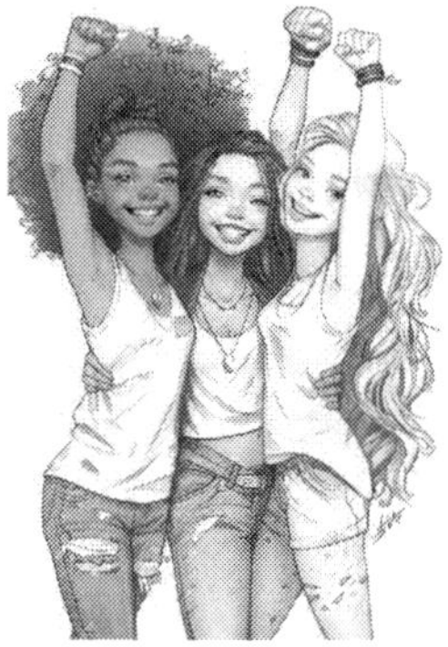

Having people you can talk to is super important. Whether it's friends, family, or even teachers, having a support system will make dealing with it easier. A solid group of friends or family members who understand what you're going through can be a game changer. Here's how to make your team even stronger:

- **Education is Power:** Sometimes, people are uncomfortable about periods because they don't understand them. Sharing what you know can help make others more supportive and understanding.
- **Find Your People:** Not everyone is comfortable talking about periods, and that's okay. Find people who are supportive and

open. They can be a great resource when you have questions or just need to let off some steam.

- **Period Parties:** Really? Yes, it's a thing. Maybe not for everybody, but I have to throw it out there. Celebrating your period is a natural part of life and can be empowering. It can be as simple as having a movie night or a small get-together with friends.
- **How to Start the Conversation:** Sometimes, being honest and straightforward is the best way to go. You might be surprised at how many people are willing to talk and share their own experiences with you.

Emotions Are Like the Weather

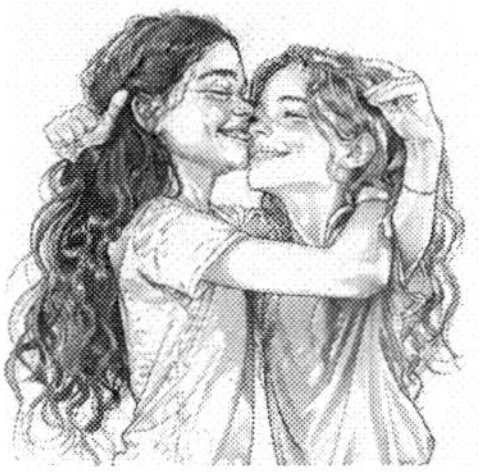

Just like the weather, your emotions can change. Recognizing and accepting your feelings can help you get through them easier. One of the most important things to remember is that it's okay to feel whatever you feel. Your emotions are real and valid, even if they seem to change at lightning speed.

- **Self-Care is Key:** Taking care of yourself is really important during your period. Whether it's watching your favorite movie, taking a warm bath, or just chilling with a book, do what makes you feel good.
- **Exercise Helps:** I know, I know, when you're feeling *blah*, the last thing you want to do is move. Even just a little exercise can help boost your mood. Dancing in your room totally counts!
- **It's Okay Not to Be Okay:** Sometimes, you need to acknowledge that you're feeling down or upset, and that's okay. You don't always have to have everything together.
- **Find What Calms You:** Whether it's meditation, writing in a

journal, or deep breathing exercises, find what helps calm you down and make that part of your routine.

<u>BONUS PRO TIP</u>:

Create a "Happy To-Do List!" Sometimes, we get so caught up in our emotions that we forget what can actually help us. I know, I've been there. Here's what you can do:

1. Create a list of happy thoughts, nice texts, and fun ideas.
2. Set an alarm on your phone to remind you to look at this list of happy things.
3. Set the alarm to go off every day of your period.
4. Title it "My Happy To-Do List!"
5. Put this list in your NOTES app.

This list is a sweet way to remind yourself of happy things. When you're feeling a little down, scroll through your list until you find something that makes you smile. By the way, this works even when you're off your period, and some people continue to use this tool when they get older.

Today is Only One Day, Tomorrow Will Be Better!

Hey, even if today totally stunk, guess what? Tomorrow's a brand new day full of new opportunities!

If things didn't go your way today—maybe you bombed a quiz, had a fallout with a friend, or your cramps totally stunk—don't sweat it! Tomorrow is a fresh start where anything can happen. It's all about keeping that hope alive.

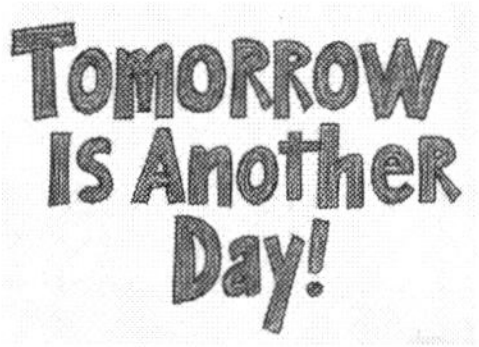

Knowing that tomorrow is there is like knowing you have a reset button in the game of life. Super powerful!

Think about all the cool stuff that can happen next in your life, like acing that test you studied for, making up with your buddy, getting the lead in the play you auditioned for, or even someday inventing the cure for cancer! Hey, it could happen!

So, toss today's emotions in the trash and get excited for a better tomorrow. Every new day is a chance to make things awesome!

Wrapping Up: Riding the Wave

Everyone who gets their period goes through these emotional ups and downs. Learning about your body, talking openly about periods, and having a support system can help make the ride a little smoother.

Coping with the sensitive side of periods can be difficult, but with the right tools and knowledge, they will help you make it through like a champ. Your feelings are valid, and it's okay to ask for help when you need it. Building a support system, getting rid of the myths, and learning to ride the wave of your emotions are all part of the journey.

ACTION TAKEAWAYS:

- Educate yourself so you know what's going on with your body.
- Talk it out with your parents and your support crew.
- Create self-care by having a well-balanced diet and exercise.
- Have some calm and kind thoughts.
- Track your moods and journal in your ***MY PERIOD POWER! WORKBOOK.***
- Create a "Happy to Do List!" in your NOTES app.
- Tomorrow is another day!

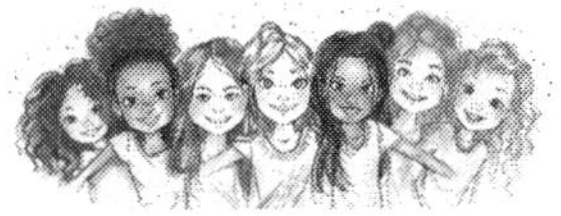

11. Make a Difference with Your Review

Remember that wild moment when you realized—"OMG! I'm growing up!" Your body was changing, your period was around the corner; a mashup of "Yikes, this is new!" and "Wow, this is so exciting!"

Think back—do you remember those whispers in the hallway about periods? You got that clueless, "Wait, a tampon goes where?" feeling? Wishing there was a guide that wasn't like a textbook or didn't sound awkward?

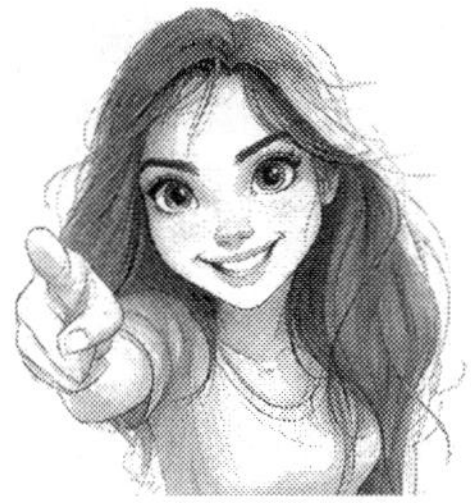

Well, guess what? You can be that guide! Yup, just like you needed advice, other teens need the same. **You** could be the one who makes them feel less alone, less confused, and way more confident.

Helping others makes you feel like a total superhero. People who lift others up live happier lives, so why not sprinkle that magic everywhere? If we have the chance to help ourselves **and** help others at the same time—well, heck—I think we should try.

Would you spend 60 seconds to make someone's life a little brighter?

1. **<u>Tap the link or scan the QR code.</u>**

<u>https://dub.sh/APPA</u>

2. **<u>Share your feelings</u>:** How did it help you? Did it make you smile? Did you have an "Oh, I get it now!" moment?

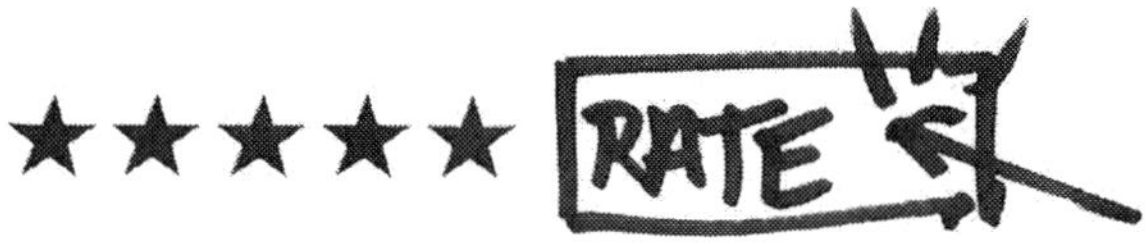

3. Give your **<u>Written Review, Your Stars</u>** ★★★★★ **<u>Rating, and Submit</u>**, and know that you just helped someone else improve their life in the coolest way possible.

4. **<u>Maybe add a picture or video</u>** of yourself along with your review and online talking about how the book helped you! I'd love to see who you are! **#MyPeriodPower!**

It feels good to share the secret sauce of growing up! So, why not be that person?

That's it! Your words could totally change someone's life! How cool is that? Thank you for being a part of this mission to spread confidence, kindness, and a whole lot of period power!

Confidence shared is confidence multiplied. Keep shining, superstar!

Your biggest fan,

SheriBelle Karper

12. Tackle Problems Like a Pro

Alright, so we've talked about the emotional ups and downs that come with periods, but what about the physical stuff? Cramps that feel like someone's doing gymnastics in your belly, bloating that makes you look like you swallowed a balloon, and other super fun stuff *(Eye roll)*. Because one minute, you're living your best life, and the next, you're wondering why you're crying over a commercial or why your stomach feels like it's hosting a WWE match. Yeah, that's your period for you. Let's figure out how to deal with these issues like the boss that you are!

Cramps: The Unwelcomed Guest

Cramps are like that annoying friend who shows up uninvited and then decides to stay way too long. They happen because your uterus is contracting to shed its lining. Sounds fun, right? Sometimes, not so much. But here's how you can show these cramps who's boss:

- **Stay Hydrated:** Drinking plenty of water might seem simple, but it's super effective. It can help ease the cramps and keep you feeling good. Sometimes, just curling up with a cup of hot raspberry leaf tea can help.

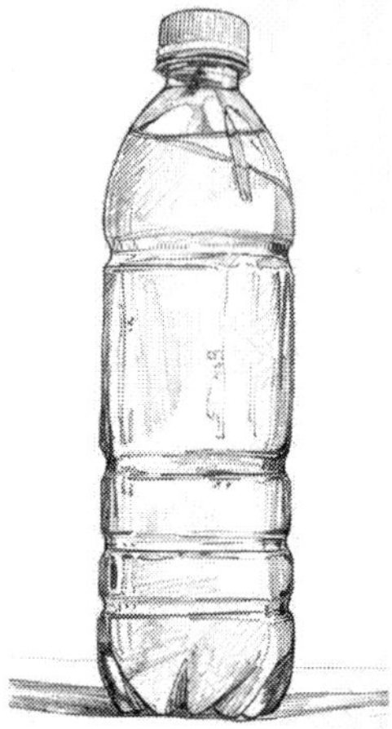

- **Heat is Your Friend:** A warm heating pad or a hot water bottle on your belly can be soothing. It's like giving your muscles a cozy hug. (**IMPORTANT:** Never sleep with a heating pad. Extended exposure to so much heat can cause burns on your skin.)
- **Move a Little:** I know, when you're feeling crampy, exercise might be the last thing on your list. But something gentle, like stretching or walking, can actually help. It's like telling your body, "Hey, let's chill out together." Some people find that yoga or stretching exercises can really help. There are specific poses that are like magic for reducing pain.
- **Over-the-Counter Pain Relief** if the pain gets really bad. Always check with an adult before taking any pills, though.

BONUS PRO TIP:

When cramps get really tough, keep a stash of Raspberry leaf tea bags. They sell them online and really work well when you drink them hot. Add a little honey if you'd like. It's a homeopathic remedy for dealing with cramps, but whatever it is, it really works for some people. I hope it works for you, too!

The Deal with Breakouts

Ever notice how your skin goes all Hollywood drama on you right before you get your period? Yeah, those breakouts aren't just random. There's another gift from our good old friend, our hormones. But just know, the guys have their own hormone wars going on, and they are going through breakouts, as well.

- **Skin Care Routine to the Rescue:** Find a gentle cleanser and stick to a simple skincare routine. Using harsh products or over-washing your skin can actually make things worse. It's like your skin is throwing a tantrum, and being gentle is the best way to calm it down.
- **Hands Off Pimples:** As tempting as it might be to pick at your skin, don't. It's like pressing a big red button that says, "Do not press!" Nothing good comes from it and can actually cause scarring.

Bloating: The Puffy Enemy

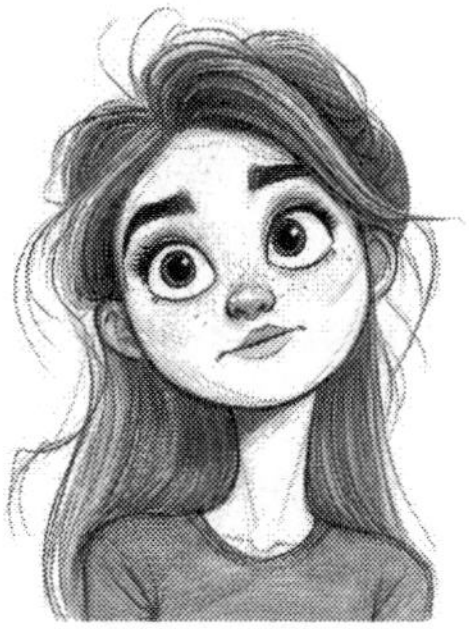

Ever feel like you could eat everything in the kitchen and still be hungry? Or that "Ugh, I feel like a balloon" feeling? Those cravings are your hormones stirring up hunger pangs. It's like they're throwing a party in your stomach but forgot to bring the food. Plus, feeling like a puffy marshmallow is another delightful part of periods for some of us, not everyone. Bloating is your body holding onto water and making you feel a little swollen. Here's how to deflate:

- **Watch What You Eat:** Eat light and avoid too much salt and sugar. Think of it like choosing characters in a video game—some foods are allies, and some foods are definitely not. Tracking it in your ***MY PERIOD POWER! WORKBOOK*** is an excellent way to track whether something is happening repeatedly. That way, you can change it.
- **Keep Sipping Water:** It sounds weird, but drinking water actually helps your body let go of excess water. It's like your body is confused and needs a reminder of what it's supposed to do.
- **Get Moving:** Again, a bit of exercise can help your body get back on track and reduce that bloated feeling.

- **Snack Smart:** Keep healthy snacks around that make you feel full, like nuts, fruits, or yogurt. It's like having your own secret stash of power-ups. Did you know certain foods can make bloating worse? Eating light, healthy meals is a good idea, and maybe saving the salty or sugary stuff for when you're feeling better.
- **Balance is Key:** Eat well-balanced meals with protein, fats, and carbs. Having a healthy diet helps keep your energy levels steady, so you don't crash and burn.

Headaches and Fatigue: The Energy Vampires

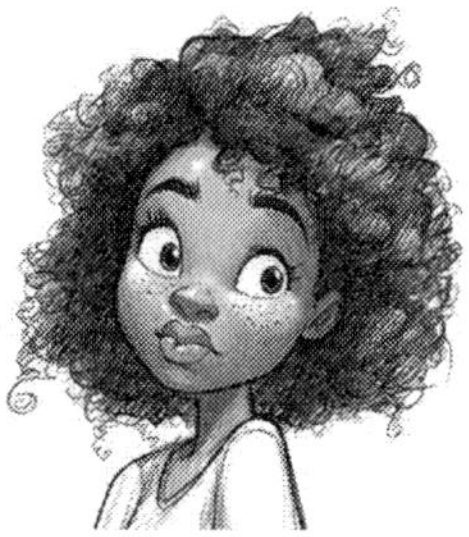

Getting a good night's sleep can be really tough when you're on your period. Between cramps, worrying about leaks, and just feeling icky, it sometimes feels like you're trying to sleep through a noisy party next door. Cramps bring along their buddies—headaches and fatigue—turning you into a walking zombie. Here's the secret to fighting these energy vampires:

- **Rest Up:** Listen to your body. If you're tired, give yourself permission to take it easy. Your body is doing a lot of work during your period, so sometimes you just need to recharge.
- **Eat Smart:** Foods high in iron and magnesium can help combat fatigue. It's like arming yourself with energy boosts throughout the day.
- **Stay Hydrated:** Yep, water is making another appearance! Staying hydrated can help keep headaches away.
- **Create a Cozy Sleep Area:** Make your room as comfy and cozy as possible. Think soft blankets, a white noise machine, or an extra pillow for hugging.
- **Sleep Routine is Your Friend:** Try to stick to a bedtime routine. Whether it is reading a book, listening to calm music,

or doing gentle stretches, find out how to signal to your body, "Hey, it's time to wind down."

The Mood Swing Survival Guide

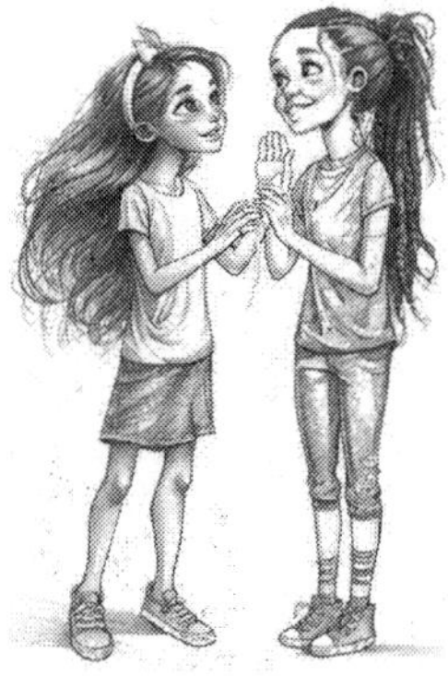

Keeping a mood diary can help you see patterns in your emotions. Also, don't underestimate the power of a good laugh. Feeling all the feels? It's totally okay. Help fix this by:

- **Talking to Friends:** "Blah, blah, blah, ha ha ha!"
- **Exercise:** Once again, exercise is a powerful cure for just about problem. Whether it's running, yoga, or shaking it out with Zumba, any kind of movement you do will help a lot.
- **Just Doing Something:** Distracting yourself by doing just about anything you love can help keep the mood monster away.
- **Funny Videos or Hanging Out with Friends:** Things that make you giggle can be just what you need.
- **Journaling:** Look out for the ***MY PERIOD POWER! WORKBOOK,*** also for sale probably wherever you bought this book, because they work perfectly together!

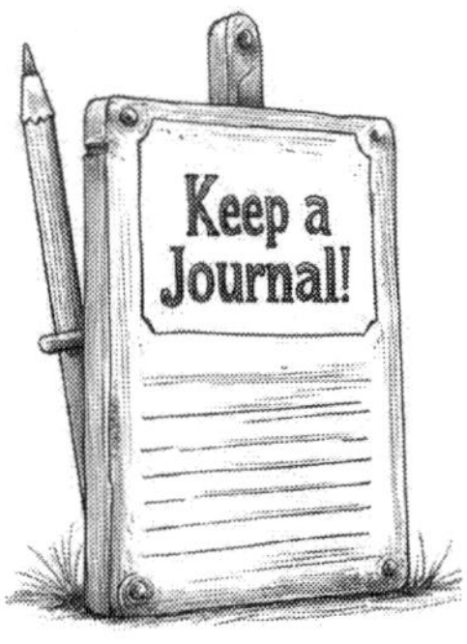

Mastering Your Menstrual Cycle

Understanding your cycle means you can figure out when your period will show up. You'll also know when you might have more energy, when you might want to eat everything in sight, and even when you might feel a bit more down than usual.

BONUS TRACKING TIPS:

Start by marking the first day of your period in your ***MY PERIOD POWER! WORKBOOK*** on the calendar or in an app. After a few months, you'll see a pattern. You might notice you always get a breakout right before your period starts or feel super energetic in the middle of your cycle. This is your body talking to you, telling you hints, so listen up!

Cycle Syncing: Some people take tracking to the next level by adjusting their activities, diet, and even social plans based on where they are in their menstrual cycle. Feeling super energetic? Maybe that's the best time to try out for the soccer team or start a big project.

Track Your Cycle Like a Pro

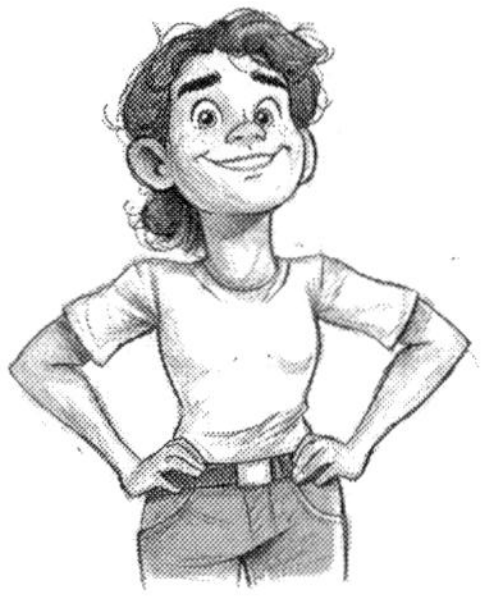

Tracking your cycle isn't about marking X's on the calendar. It's about knowing your body and all its signals. Writing it all down is like talking to your own personal assistant. Your workbook can help you figure out when your period is going to start, when you're ovulating (a.k.a. prime pimple time—thanks, hormones. (Uuuugh)). It can even remind you when to get snacks and pads, so there's no last-minute screaming, "Hey mom! We need to go to the store NOW!" It's like having a secret diary that whispers, "Psssst, your period is coming. Grab the stash!"

Leak-Proof Strategies

Even with the right absorbency, leaks can happen, especially at night or during sports. Here are some pro tips to help steer clear of any embarrassing moments:

- **Double Up:** For extra protection, consider wearing a tampon and a pad OR a menstrual cup and a pad.
- **Right Fit:** Make sure your underwear fits snugly. This helps your pad stay in place and provides backup in case of leaks.
- **Period Panties:** These are a game-changer. They are designed to be super absorbent, so even if you do have a leak, these panties have you covered.

When Periods Feel Like Too Much

Sometimes, even with all the tips and tricks, it can still feel overwhelming. It's okay to have those moments when you're "*just over it.*" Here's what to do:

- **Talk It Out:** Sometimes, talking about how much periods stink can make you feel a little better.
- **Give Yourself a Break:** It's okay to have a day where you're not 100%. Sometimes, the best thing you can do is acknowledge that you're doing the best you can.

Wrapping It All Up on Period Products

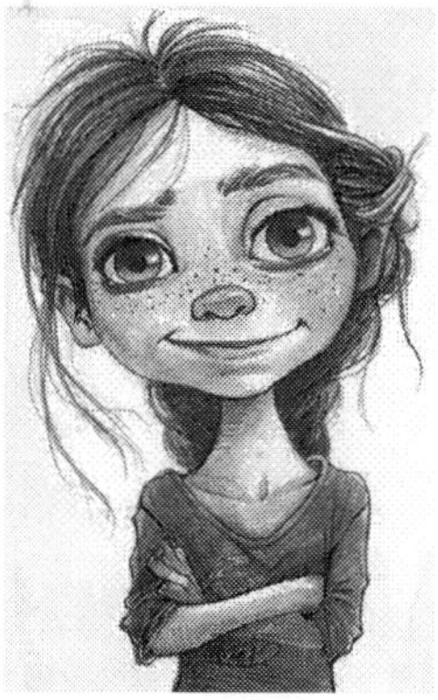

Okay, Sunshine! Whew! That was a lot of information! There's a lot of physical stuff to get used to, I know. Just take it slow and easy. No rush to get into tampons or even menstrual cups. Whether you use pads, tampons, menstrual cups, or a combination of the three, when you're ready, you can rock your period like the queen you are. Everything is based on your decision timeline. You've got this!

When to Call In the Pros

Sometimes, despite all your best efforts, period problems can feel like too much to handle. If your cramps are super severe, or if anything else about your period feels way off, it's okay (and really important) to talk to a doctor or trusted adult. It's like calling in the troops when you're dealing with a tough villain.

Wrap-Up: You've Got This!

Dealing with the signs and the physical hints that come with periods can feel like a battle, but you now have some pretty awesome tools to fight back. You're not alone in this. Talk it out with your parents, an older sibling, your bestie, your teacher, school nurse, or your doctor. You have many options, so please reach out!

ACTION TAKEAWAYS:

- Cramps—heat, exercise, and hydration.
- Wash your face and don't pop pimples.
- Watch what you eat and have a balanced diet to avoid bloating.
- It's okay to combine period products.
- Make your bed cozy and comfortable for a good rest.
- Talk it out with your parents, your support crew, and your doctor, if necessary. You are not alone.

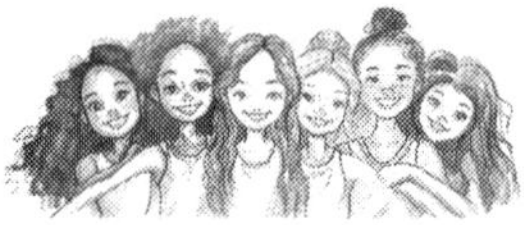

13. Short Chapter About Grooming.... (Short, But Important!)

While we're on the subject of taking care of ourselves, here are some extra pro moves to keep you on the good side of periods.

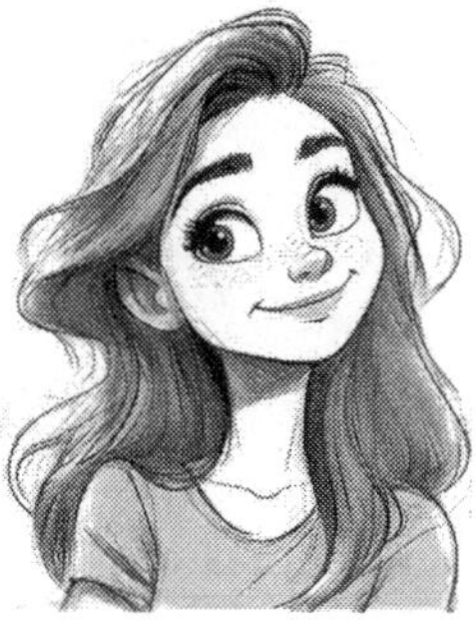

Hey Honey, Take a Shower Already! (No, Seriously, Take a Shower!)

I probably don't need to say it, because my period crew here is so in tune with their bodies, but hey, I can't skip something this important.

Whether you like it or not, when our bodies change, these changes can sometimes come with odors. (Yuuuck!) Yes, I said it. I had to! Just like I would tell you if you had spinach in your teeth, we're in this together, and since we're together, I'd like you to be standing next to me *and* smelling good.

And, maybe someone bought you some **deodorant or antiperspirant** recently. Yeah, smelling good doesn't just stop with soap and water. Very soon, it will become quite clear who at school *does* or *doesn't* use deodorant! (Eeeeek! Stink City!) You'll probably want to be the one that smells like a "Spring Meadow" or feels "Powder Fresh!" so people will want to sit with you at lunch! Using a deodorant or an antiperspirant is your secret weapon to keep you smelling fresh and clean, even during a hard workout!

And while we're at it, it might not hurt to get a mirror and check out what you've got down there. Yeah, *that* down there. Yes, take a look at your vulva (that's the outside area down there). (Whaaat???!!!) Yeah, I know—weird! Well, yes, and no. Yes, because you've probably never taken a peek at that before, but no (not weird), because it's your super cool body, and why should your body be weird, right? I'm not saying to gaze at it for hours! Hahahaha! All I'm saying is, take a peek and look at all the players. This is your body, and no one has to know.

Whew! Back to Grooming!

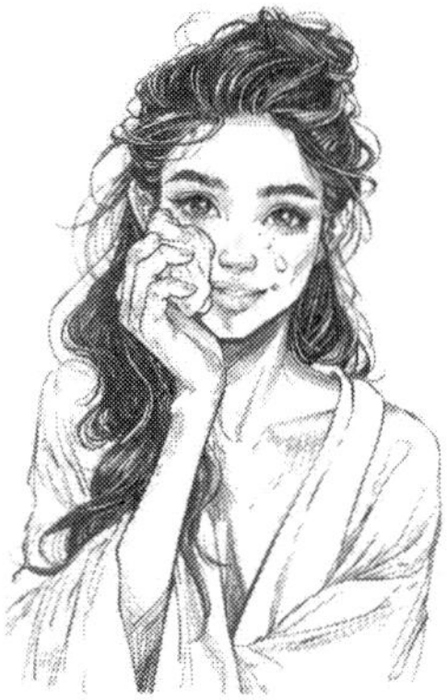

- **During Your Period You Need to Take a Shower Every Day:** This includes washing your "down there," inside your butt-crack (did I just say that?!) and under your armpits—with soap! And, of course, rinse everything thoroughly.
- **Always Wash Your Hands** before and after dealing with your period stuff. It's like putting on armor against germy enemies.
- **Wash Your Face:** Find a gentle, non-drying cleanser and stick to a simple skincare program of washing morning and night.
- **Moisturize!** See "1" and "2" below about building a skincare routine to keep your face fresh and help get rid of those darn pimples.

1. ***Morning*****:** After you wash your face in the morning, apply a moisturizing sunscreen with at least SPF 30. Try to make sure that it's oil free, and the bottle should say "non-comedogenic," which is big talk for "won't clog your pores."

2. ***Nighttime*****:** After you wash your face at night, make sure that you follow it up with a light moisturizer that does NOT have an SPF factor. We want you to have a clean, light lotion that is oil free and, once again, non-comedogenic.

Once you stick to this schedule of washing and moisturizing twice a day, every day, you will notice a big difference in your skin. You look even more adorable, and trust me, you'll thank me!

Don't Pop Those Pimples!

No matter how tempting, don't pop your pimples. Doing this can push gunk deeper into your skin and even lead to scars. Taking care of your skin will help keep it clear and happy so that you can feel more confident.

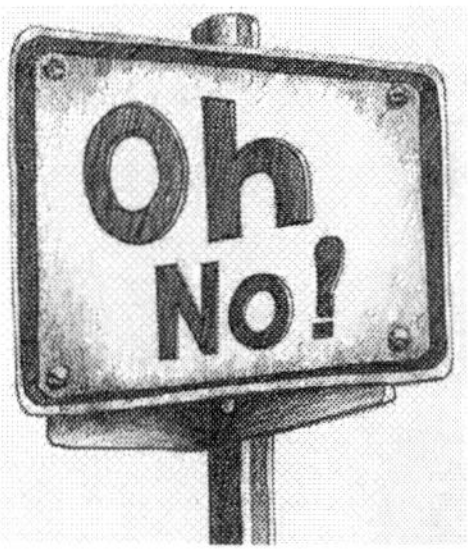

BONUS PRO TIP:

If you have a giant zit that won't go away, try this emergency idea. Have one of your parents stop by the drugstore or store and pick up a tube of WHITE toothpaste or Benzoyl Peroxide paste. Make sure to get the old-school kind that looks like a white paste —NOT the gel kind. Once you get it, wash your face well, pat it dry, and put a blob of the paste on the big zit only, not on the skin surrounding the zit. Let it sit there for a long time, like an hour. Yes, I said hour! Hide out in your room, if you have to! This trick may help to dry out the gunk inside the zit below the skin's surface. It also sort of sterilizes the little "infection" brewing below the surface that's creating the zit. Only try it on one pimple first, and see how your skin reacts. DO NOT put either paste all over your face. It could irritate your skin and give you a red rash! (Aaaaargh!) You don't want a red face of irritation! This tip is only for occasional use on a giant zit. It doesn't work for everyone, so good luck! I hope it works for you!

DOUBLE BONUS PRO TIP:

If you had acne scarring before reading this book (because now you know you're not supposed to pick at your blemishes), sunscreen also helps protect those scars from turning dark. Once they turn dark, they will eventually fade, but it takes a really long time. So why not stop the process and wear sunscreen so they won't get dark!

TRIPLE BONUS PRO TIP:

If you feel like your blemishes are really out of control and you're sticking to a regular skincare system of washing and applying lotion morning and night, your first stop is to see a dermatologist. After a while, if the dermatologist's ideas don't seem to help, you might see an endocrinologist (whoa, that's a lot of letters!), which is a doctor that deals with—go ahead and guess—they deal with hormones! Yeah, those pesky hormones could be at play. But going to see an endocrinologist is really only if you have an extreme acne problem.

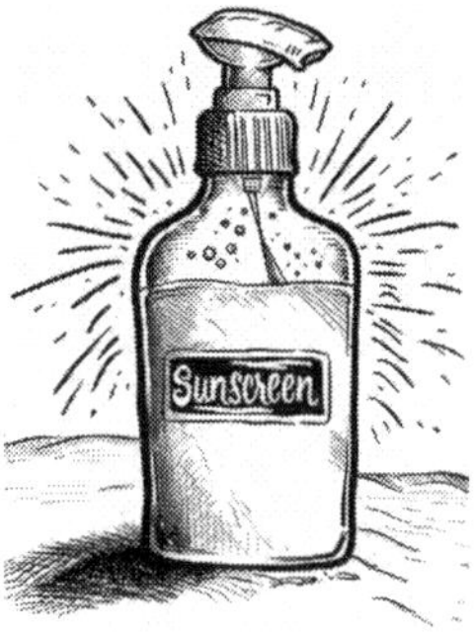

Sunscreen is Your Bestie

First up, sunscreen is a must all over your body. Not just any sunscreen, but one with a high SPF. SPF stands for Sun Protection Factor: This tells you how well the sunscreen can keep your skin safe from UVA and UVB rays (those are what burn you). If you have fair skin, you'll need an even higher SPF because your skin is super sensitive to the sun. I recommend nothing less than SPF 30, but SPF 50 is even better.

You should test different sunscreens to figure out which one's feel good on your skin. I recommend a moisturizing sunscreen.

Re-Apply Like a Pro

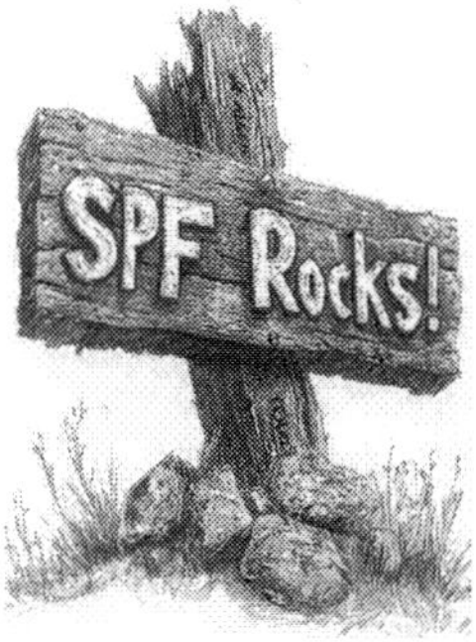

Slapping on sunscreen isn't just a once-and-done deal. You've got to reapply it every couple of hours. And if you're diving into the pool or catching waves at the beach, it's important to put it on again as soon as you dry off and towel off. Water washes away sunscreen, and even the "water-resistant" types don't stick around forever.

Here's the lowdown on this chapter: This bathing and grooming thing? Yeah, it's a forever kind of deal, okay? It's all about taking care of yourself, listening to your body, and letting other people help you along the way.

That's it, baby! I told you it was short!

<u>**ACTION TAKEAWAYS:**</u>

- You need to shower and wash your entire body daily. Rinse everything well.
- Get some nice smelling deodorant or antiperspirant.
- You need to wash your face twice a day. In the shower is OK!
- Use great moisturizers with SPF 50+ during the day and a calming moisturizer for nighttime.
- Don't pick at your pimples or blackheads on your face.
- If your acne becomes extreme, get in touch with the right doctors.

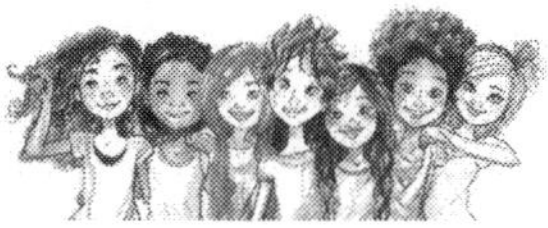

14. Your Body is Changing

Ever feel like you went to bed one size and woke up another? It's totally weird, but also totally normal. Everybody goes through it —guys, girls, and everyone in between. And that means that your body is doing exactly what it's meant to do—grow up! This chapter is all about your ever-changing body, figuring out what's happening, and totally rocking those big changes!

Welcome to your teen years! This is when your body starts a project that's kind of like a major room makeover! It's called puberty! Here are a couple of things you can expect:

Growth Spurts

Have you noticed that one day your pants fit, and the next day they're like capris? You might suddenly feel like your body is stretching faster than cheese on a pizza.

We're talking about growth spurts. It's totally natural for your body to suddenly kick into high gear and shoot up a couple of inches during your teen years. This happens because your body is getting all the right signals from your brain to grow, grow, grow!

If you're eating more or feeling like your shoes are suddenly too tight, you're right on target. You need to get bigger because you don't want to stay like a kid-sized candy bar your whole life, right? All these things are part of the giant plan of growing up.

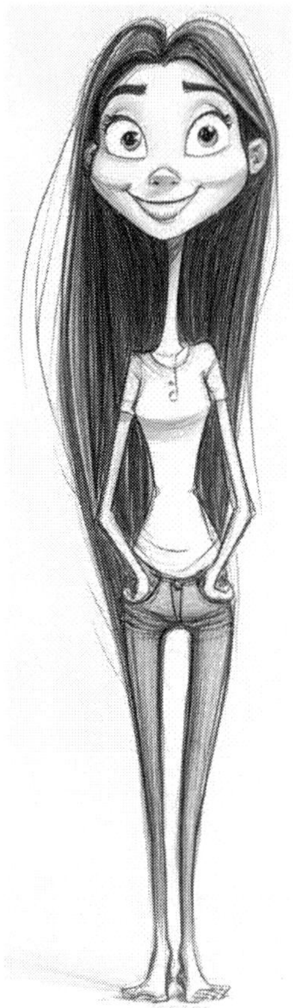

During these growth spurts, you might feel a bit clumsy or awkward. Imagine a puppy growing into its paws! Yep, that's you! Your arms and legs might grow faster than the rest of you, making you feel a little gangly. Don't sweat it, though. Everyone goes through this phase. It's just your body trying to figure out how to handle its new size and strength. It's a great excuse if you're suddenly tripping over your feet more than usual!

The coolest part? Growth spurts mean you're getting closer to becoming the adult version of you. It's exciting to see the changes, even if they sometimes feel a bit weird. Make sure you're eating right and getting plenty of sleep because your body is doing a ton of work at night to get taller and stronger. And hey, always remember to stretch and stay active. It helps make those growing muscles and bones strong and flexible.

Curves Are Cool!

As you grow up, you might notice that your body is curving out here and there. Your body is basically sculpting itself into its new, grown-up shape! It's like your body's way of preparing for all the amazing things you will do as an adult. Whether it's your hips getting a bit wider or your chest is starting to develop, these changes are about becoming the unique version of YOU!

It's okay to feel a little weird about your body changing. Everybody grows at their own pace and in their own way. If you or your friends develop curves at different times and at different speeds. It's no biggie, it's just how bodies work. Curves are great because they're a sign that your body is doing all the behind-the-scenes magic to make sure you're healthy and strong.

Enjoy these changes by wearing clothes that feel good and fit your style. Clothes can boost your confidence, especially when your body starts to look different. Maybe it's time to go shopping! (Yes, please) Find outfits that make you feel awesome and embrace your new shape in a way that makes you smile.

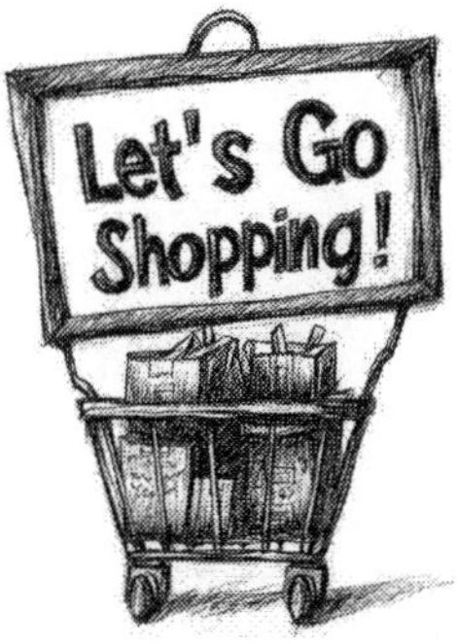

So celebrate your curves—they're part of the incredible person you are becoming!

ACTION TAKEAWAYS:

- Shooting up a couple of inches during puberty is completely normal.
- Try to get enough rest, because a lot of puberty action happens at night when you sleep. Make sure you're eating a balanced diet. Your body needs good food right now.
- Go shopping for some new clothes that fit your new shape and make you feel confident. Make sure that it's a style that makes you smile!
- Find out more about your body changes in the companion book, ***MY BODY POWER!*** sold where you found this book.
- Got questions? Talk it out with your parents or a trusted adult.

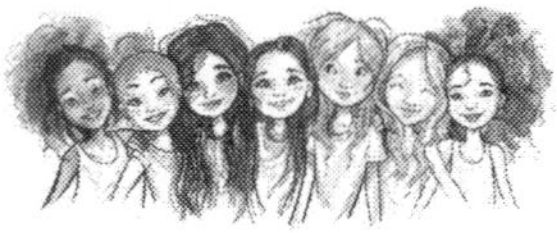

15. Now I Have to Face the World?... Face It Like a Boss!

Yes, You Can Do This!

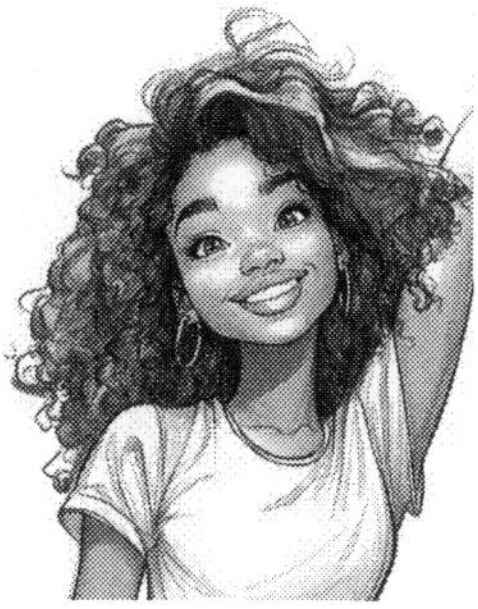

Now you have the basics down. You know how to cope with cramps, and you're pretty much a pro at handling the emotional ups and downs, but what about when you have to face the world? School, sports, sleepovers—oh, my! Let's break down how to manage your period when you're out there living your best life and get into the nitty-gritty of making your period less of a big deal when you're doing, well, anything.

Dealing With Period Emergencies

What happens if you're caught off guard? Maybe you forgot your period kit, or your period decided to surprise you at the worst possible time.

- **DIY Protection:** No pad or tampon? Ask a friend! Or if you're in school, sometimes the nurse's office has spares. In a real pinch, rolling up toilet paper as a temporary pad can save the day. It's not perfect, but it will work until you can get the real deal.
- **Stain SOS!:** If you get a stain on your clothes, tie a hoodie or sweater around your waist to cover your backside. It's a classic move—even I had to do it. Cold water and soap can also help get rid of stains quickly if you can sneak away to a bathroom. However, never use hot water because it sets the stain and makes it difficult to get out.

How to Chat About It Without Freaking Out

Talking about your period shouldn't be a big deal, but sometimes it feels like it is. Here's how to make it less awkward:

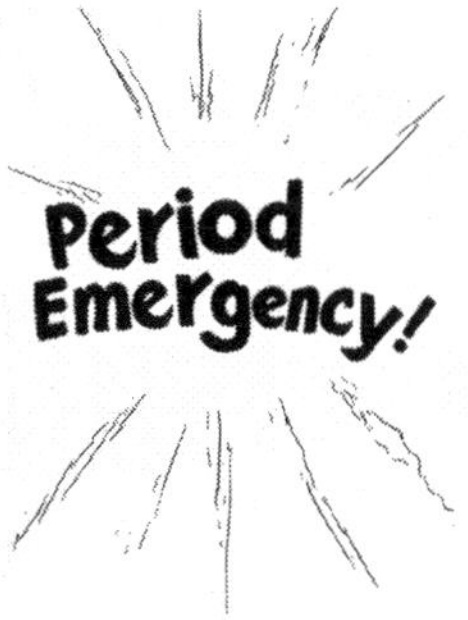

- **Just Say It:** Honestly, the more chill you are about it, the less of a big deal it becomes. Practice by saying "period" out loud without whispering. Like, "I'm on my period," or "I'm having a period emergency!" It's a natural thing, after all.
- **Educate Your Friends:** Got friends who are clueless about periods or think they're gross? A little education goes a long way. Share cool facts about how periods are a sign of good health.

<u>**INTERESTING FACT**</u>**:**

Did you know that if someone is extremely unhealthy, or a seriously intense athlete, or in a super high-stress situation, their period probably won't come or will be very irregular? That's because their body is trying to protect a potential baby. It doesn't want a baby to be born into an unhealthy situation or a high-stress environment. Your body naturally knows. Isn't that amazing? That's why some seriously hardcore athletes don't have regular periods until they have slowed their practice and sports schedule. This usually only happens during super intense training—like Olympic-level athletes—not just on your school's team (like soccer or cheer squad). It only happens in highly repetitive and drastic situations. The body is an incredible thing! Super cool!

When You're Not Feeling It

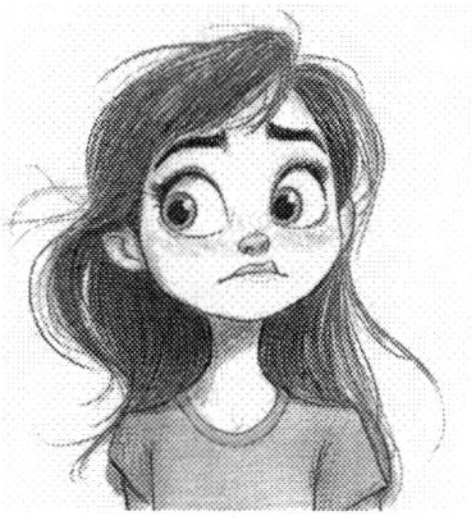

There will be days when your period makes you feel like canceling all your plans and just hibernating. And you know what? That's totally okay.

- **Listen to Your Body:** If you're not up for something, it's okay to say no. Your body is doing a lot right now. Sometimes, rest is what you need. So, take care of that beautiful body! (Just make sure that you're canceling because of real issues, not just because you want to avoid something.)
- **Self-Care Sundays (or Any Day):** Make self-care a priority, especially during your period. Bubble baths, your favorite movies, or just doodling in your notebook can be perfect for lifting your spirits.

BONUS PRO TIP:

Write down the difficult days in your ***MY PERIOD POWER! WORKBOOK*** so that maybe you can start noticing a pattern of which days of your period you need the most self-care. That way, you can organize your schedule a little or prepare yourself mentally to plan for that rough second day, or that heavier flow third day. Whatever schedule your body tells you is repeating, you can figure this out in your workbook. We're working together to make this easier for you!

Periods and Sports: The Confidence Game

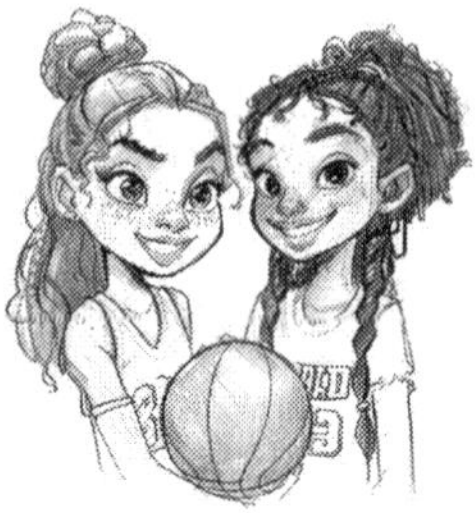

Playing sports when you're on your period can feel extra challenging, but it's totally doable. The key is being prepared. Sports on your period is actually a good thing, because exercise releases *endorphins*, which are like natural painkillers and mood lifters.

- **Pick Your Protection:** If you're into sports, tampons or menstrual cups might be more your speed. They stay in place better when you're running, jumping, or swimming.
- **Wear Black Shorts or Pants:** They're great for hiding leaks and give you that extra bit of confidence.
- **Wear What Works:** Wear gear that makes you feel secure. There are even workout leggings designed for periods.
- **Check Your Gear:** Before a big game or practice, double-check that you have everything you need to manage your period. It's like packing an extra snack, just in case.

Sonia Told Me Her First Period Story

"I remember the day when my period started before my biggest soccer match of the season. I know, it was only a co-ed game, but we were all so competitive, and it was really important to me. My heart sank when I went to go pee and I saw blood in my underwear. I totally panicked. I was the striker for the team, and I was known for my speed and strength. But right then, I felt powerless.

"The thought of playing that game on my first period was freaking me out. I was scared the boys would notice and make fun of me. Or worse, that I wouldn't be able to play my best. I thought about sitting out the game, but I couldn't stand the thought of letting my team down.

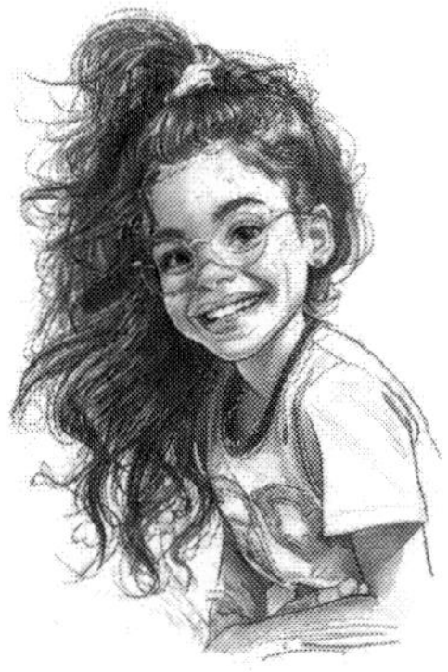

"I told my coach, and she gave me some advice. She was like a ray of hope when I felt like I was losing my mind. She gave me a big pep talk saying things like, 'You've got this!' She gave me a pad to wear and some extras to put in my gym bag. She gave me a high-five and told me, 'Get out there!' I ran out on the field, totally filled with nerves and excitement.

"I was super surprised when the match went on like any other game. The boys on the team were so focused on winning that they didn't notice a thing. My fears disappeared as I chased that ball down the field. My heart exploded when I scored the winning goal! I was so proud of myself! Not just for winning, but for getting rid of all of those fears. It was a fantastic day!"

Periods and Swimming: Making a Splash

Worried about swimming when you're on your period? Don't be. With the right protection, you can totally dive in without any stress.

- **Tampons and Menstrual Cups:** These are your best friends for swimming because they're worn internally. Remember: It's important to change your tampon or empty your cup promptly after you're finished swimming.
- **Dark-Colored Swimwear:** Just like in sports, dark colors can help you feel more secure, just in case.

School Daze: Periods in the Classroom

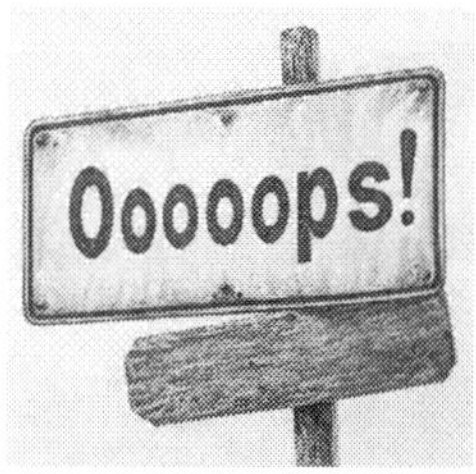

I know it feels like a minefield when you're on your period. What if you leak? What if you need to change your pad or tampon during class? Here are some answers:

- **Period Kit to the Rescue:** Keep a little bag with pads, tampons, or whatever you use, along with some spare undies in your backpack. It's like your secret weapon.
- **Buy a zippered, non-see-through pouch,** just in case it falls out of your backpack, then you won't be embarrassed.
- **Know the Code:** Figure out a secret sign or "code word" with your friends or teacher if you need to make a quick exit. "Can I borrow a pencil?" can be your undercover message for "I need to deal with period stuff."

Sleepovers and Camps: The Overnight Challenge

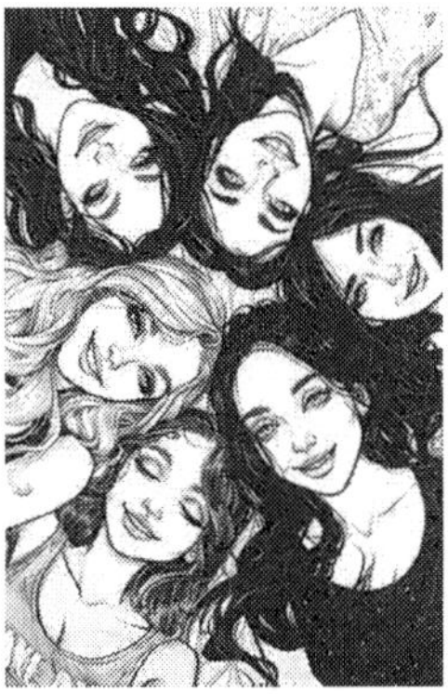

Sleeping away from home means planning ahead—whether it's a sleepover at a friend's house or an overnight at a campground—you've got this.

- **Pack Extra Supplies:** Bring more period products than you think you'll need. It's better to have too much than not enough. And, who knows, maybe one of your sleepover buds might need to borrow something.
- **Have a Plan:** Talk to your friend or a teacher you trust about where you can store your period supplies, and where you can change them in privacy.

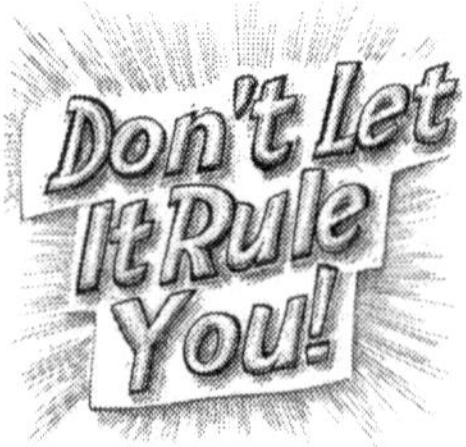

Wrapping It All Up: Periods Don't Rule You

See? With a little prep and some insider knowledge, you can totally handle your period no matter where or what you're doing. It's all about planning ahead and having back-ups, just in case. And even if you're caught off-guard, you'll probably have someone to help you manage. Getting through life with your period is totally doable, and it doesn't have to be a drag. Whether you're in school, hanging out with friends, playing co-ed soccer, or hitting the pool, you have the power to manage your period like the champ you are.

Having your period is simply a part of life. It shouldn't stop you from doing anything you love or hanging out with your friends. You are way stronger and more prepared than you think.

Everyone's period experience is different, so what works for one person might not work for another. The key is to find what makes your period easier for you. You're not alone in this. You've got a whole squad of people who get it, even if it doesn't always feel like it.

Coming up next, we're tackling how to deal with guys… yeah, that!

ACTION TAKEAWAYS:

- Buy a zippered fabric pouch that is not see-through to store your backpack period kit.
- Prepare your period kit and tuck it in your backpack.
- Buy black pants, black shorts, black leggings, black swimsuit, and/or black underwear to help hide leaks if they happen.
- Practice saying "period" and period phrases out loud.
- Create codewords and make back-up plans with friends and adults for emergencies.
- Track your period!
- Let your parents be a part of this transition. They can help you find the strength to face the world head on!

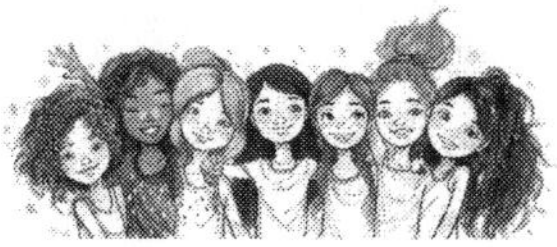

16. Decoding Guys, Giggles, and Getting Real

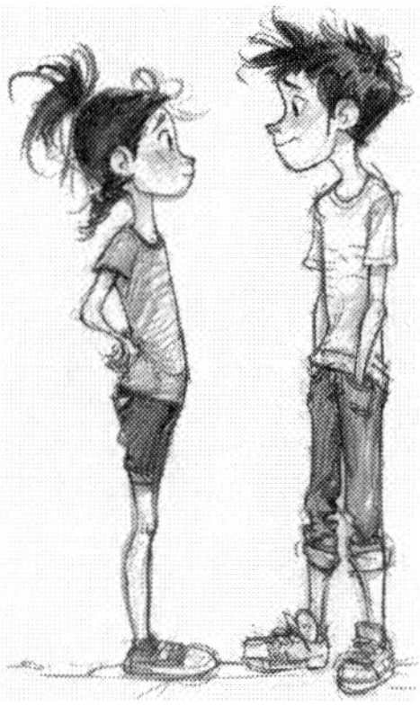

Alright squad, get ready because we're about to dive deep into the Bermuda Triangle of being a teenager—guys understanding (or not understanding) periods. It's like navigating a minefield with your eyes closed. But don't worry, I've got your back. Let's embrace the awkward, the funny, and the downright face-palm moments that come with guys and period talk.

But wait just a minute! When did boys become guys? Yes, boys are changing, too. One day, they're boys, and the next day, they are guys. They will look different, sound different, and act different because somehow, somewhere, they turned into—well, guys! It's important to know that everybody is changing right now, even the guys.

The Comedy Central of Jokes (O.T.R. Does Not Mean "One Terrific Redhead")

You've probably noticed that some boys think they're stand-up comedians when it comes to period jokes. "Is it shark week?" they chuckle, thinking they've just cracked some radical comedy code. Or the classic, "Hide the chocolate—she's on the warpath!" Like somehow, your period turns you into Godzilla on a cocoa bean hunt. I mean, really? *(Eye roll)* And by the way, O.T.R. stands for *"on the rag."* Not nice, I know. But you need to know what the codes mean so you're not caught off guard. I've got to keep you prepared.

Here's the scoop: Most of the time, these guys aren't trying to be mean. They're just a bit clueless, or even nervous. It's like they've learned everything they know about periods from bad comedy shows, but that doesn't mean you've got to let it slide.

BONUS PRO TIP:

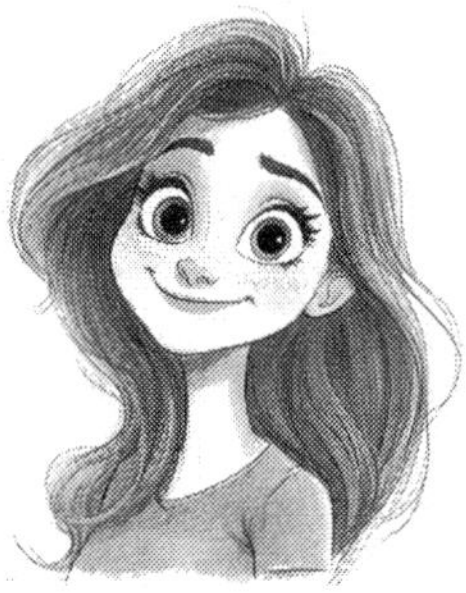

- **Try to Be Funny Right Back!** A little humor goes a long way in making sensitive subjects like this a little less sensitive. If you're feeling sassy, a "Wow, did you come up with that all by yourself?" is a great reaction.
- **The Joke's on Who?** Okay, we've all heard them, those jokes about periods that some guys think are the height of comedy. "Are you on your period or something?" As if that explains every mood ever. Or the classic, "Watch out, she's PMS-ing!" It seems like they say this anytime a girl has an opinion. (Ugghh!)

For me, I always tried to respond with something kind of funny, but you do you!

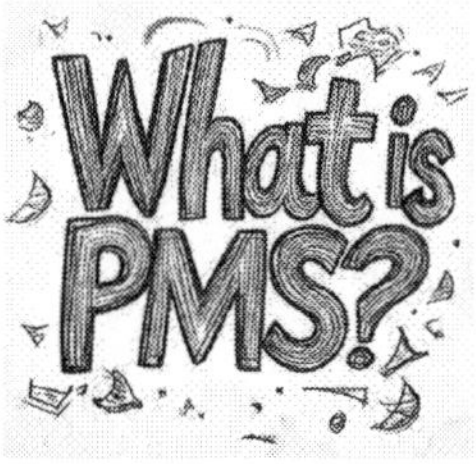

What is PMS?

PMS stands for Premenstrual Syndrome. It's a bunch of symptoms that some girls and women have to deal with about a week before their period. It's a combination of moodiness, hunger, tiredness, and emotions—It's a mash-up of all the crummiest parts of having your period.

Cringe-Fest 101: The Awkward Silence

Have you ever mentioned your period around a boy and watched him squirm like he was suddenly in the hot seat on a game show? Yeah, that's called the "awkward silence"—when boys act like you've just spoken in an alien tongue, the room goes quiet, and you can practically hear the crickets.

- **Behind the Awkwardness:** Truth bomb—it's all about the unknown. For a lot of guys, knowing that girls have a period is like exploring the dark side of the moon. They know it exists, but what's really going on there? Who knows?!
- **The Friendship Move:** If you're feeling up for it, helping to demystify your period can be kind of empowering. Sharing basics like, "It's just a natural body process, dude, not a curse," can help normalize it. Who knows, you might just enlighten someone.
- **Bridge Building:** If you're feeling brave, shedding some light on the subject can turn awkwardness into understanding. "Hey, it's just a natural thing that happens to half the population. No biggie." Sometimes, a little info can go a long way, making everyone feel more comfortable.

Everyone's a bit awkward about stuff they don't understand. A lot of guys think periods are like the final frontier of mysteries—meaning they just don't want to know about it. They know what happens, but the details? A total fog. And, some of them want to keep it that way. Also, maybe they're not even ready to talk about their own puberty, much less find out anything about yours.

The Good Guys Get It

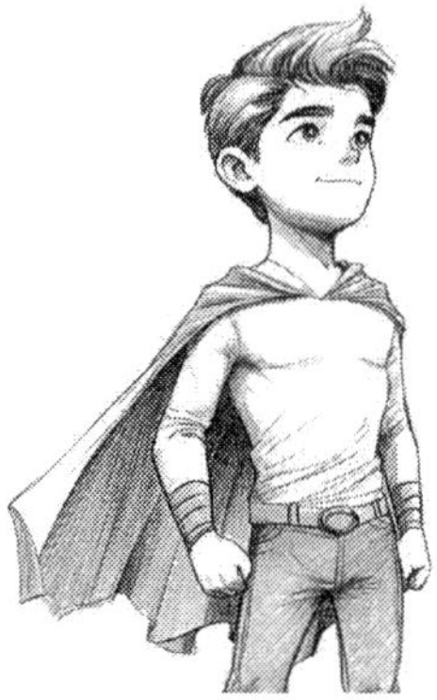

Not all heroes wear capes, and not all boys are clueless or awkward about periods. Some guys are totally on board and get that it's a part of life. These are the ones who aren't embarrassed to help you buy tampons or get why you might not be up for swimming. Here's to the guys who understand that periods are a part of life and don't make it weird.

- **Shout Out to the Allies:** These dudes are the real MVPs. They listen, they learn, and they don't make a big deal out of it. If you've got friends like this, give them a mental high-five. They're setting the bar nice and high for how everyone else should be.
- **Props to These Guys:** They're the real deal—respectful, informed, and totally unfazed. They're proof that with a bit of understanding and empathy, periods don't have to be a big deal.
- **Boyfriends or Significant Others:** At some point in your life, you'll have someone special (maybe even now), and they'll need to understand what you're going through. It's important to talk with that special person to let them know why you're having a bad day or why you are supercharged with extra energy. You don't want them to be like, "Whoa! Who *is* this?" You want them to be like, "Oh, okay… I got you!"

Game Plan for Navigating Period Talk with Guys

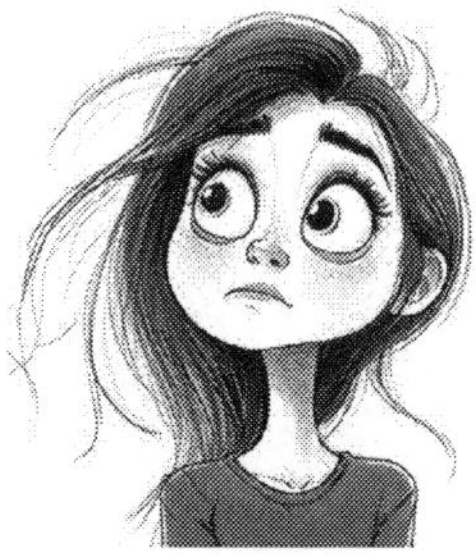

Mastering the art of period talk with boys is like learning to ride a bike—a bit wobbly at first, but totally doable with some practice.

- **You're the Boss:** You decide how much you want to share about your period. If someone is being cool, and you feel like sharing, awesome. If not, that's cool, too. Your body, your rules.
- **Knowledge is Power:** Dropping some period knowledge bombs (gently, of course) can change the game. It's hard to make weird jokes about something you understand. Helping guys understand periods better can turn awkward jokes into respectful conversations.
- **Laugh It Off:** Sometimes, laughing together is the best way to break the ice. If you can joke about your period in a way that's comfortable for you, it can make the whole topic less awkward. If all else fails, a sense of humor can be your best defense.

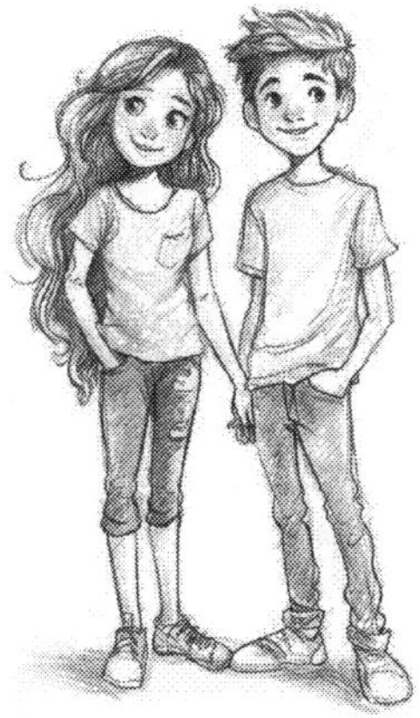

The Final Word: Periods, Guys, and Moving Forward

There you have it: Your insider's guide to dealing with guys about period talk. Whether you're dealing with jokesters, the awkward squad, or the cool allies, you're helping pave the way for a future where periods are just another part of life, not a secret source of embarrassment.

Keep being your confident self. Share your stories, and maybe, just maybe, get to a place where period talk is no big deal for anyone. Keep shining, keep educating, and let's keep the conversation going. Together, we're unstoppable!

Coming up next, we're taking on how to shift your mindset from "My period, ugh" to "I've got this!" It's all about finding and using your period power to fuel your awesome self. Get ready to turn that period pain into period pride!

ACTION TAKEAWAYS:

- Create a funny comeback and have it ready to go. Practice it! Make it your own so you won't stumble through the words when you need them!
- High-five the good guys!
- Talk to your parents and your older siblings about how they handled awkward moments like these. Some of your conversations about this might be hysterical!

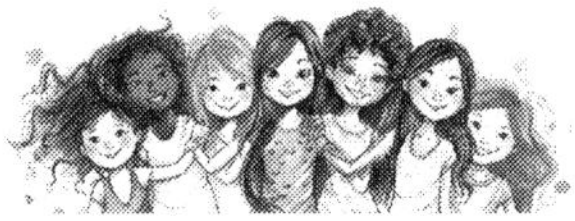

17. Finding Your Period Power!

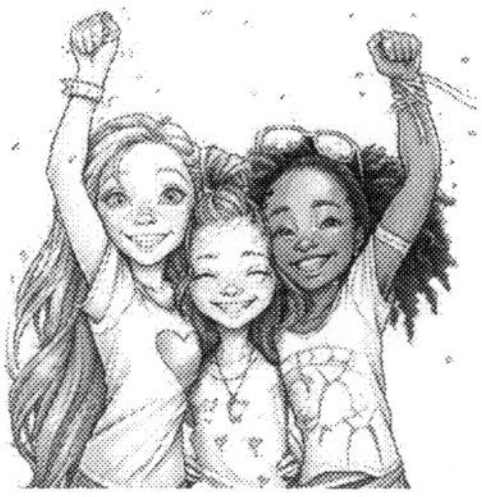

Now we've started to shift the vibe from "Ugh, why me?" to "My period stinks" to "Okay, I've got this!" But how do you start feeling proud of something that's mostly been a pain, and turn it into "My period is actually kind of cool." Sound impossible? Stick with me here—it's all about attitude and action, and believe it or not, a little bit of fun.

Embrace Period Positivity

Let's talk about flipping the script on how we see our periods. Yeah, they can be a pain (literally), but they're also a sign that your body is doing its thing and keeping you healthy.

- **Periods are Powerful:** Having a period means your body's working like it's supposed to. It's a sign of good health and that you're growing up. That's pretty amazing when you think about it.

- **Celebrate the Milestones:** Getting your period is a big deal when you're growing up. It's okay to treat it that way. Some cultures even have celebrations. You don't need to throw a party, but acknowledging this step in your life can be empowering.

Cool Ways To Celebrate Your Cycle

Having your period is a natural, healthy part of life. So, why not find fun ways to enjoy it, or at least not dread it?

- **Party Packs:** Create a little celebration kit for yourself each month. Fill it with your favorite treats, a new book, or even some interesting new period products. It's like a birthday party every month, but for your uterus!
- **Movie Marathon:** Pick a weekend during your period for a movie marathon. Invite friends over and enjoy some time with all your favorite flicks. Make it a theme—like strong female leads—choose anything you like!

Breaking the Silence: Talking About Periods

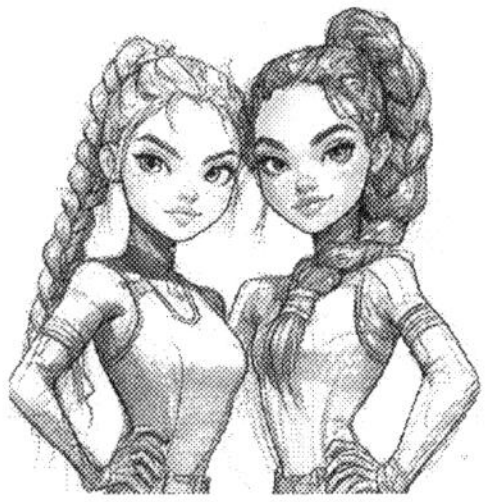

One of the best ways to feel more positive about your period is to get comfortable talking about it. The more we talk, the less weird it feels.

- **Period Chats:** Start conversations with your friends about periods. You'll be surprised how many people feel relieved to talk about it openly. It's like opening the floodgates to share experiences and support.
- **Educate and Spread the Word:** Learn as much as possible about periods and share that knowledge. Whether it's correcting misconceptions or sharing tips, every little bit helps

break down the stigma.

- **Be a Period Myth Buster!:** Be ready to correct any misinformation when you hear it. Do you have friends who think they can't swim during their period? Educate them! It's like being a superhero for period truth.
- **Book Club:** Start a book club with your best buds, focused on books about puberty and menstruation. It's a way to learn, laugh, and talk about experiences in a safe space.

Speaking Up: Period Projects and Presentations

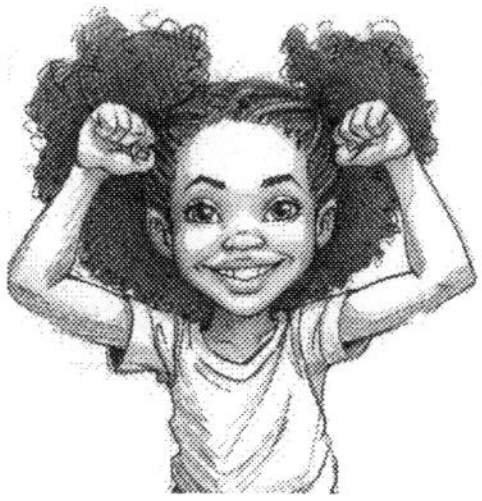

- **Science Fair, Period Style:** Do a science project on menstruation. You could cover everything from the history of period products to how different cultures view menstruation. It's a great way to educate and break the ice.
- **Art for Awareness:** Use art to express and share the experience. It could be a painting, a digital piece, or even a comic strip. Art is a powerful way to communicate and can help others feel seen and understood.

Using Your Voice for Goodness

Feeling empowered about your period also means recognizing that not everyone has the same access to products or education.

- **Period Product Drive:** Organize a period product drive at your school. Collect pads, tampons, and menstrual cups for those in need within your community. Helping others less fortunate than yourself is a beautiful thing.
- **Take Action:** Learn about period poverty and begin the conversation with your school or community leaders. Could

your school provide free period products in bathrooms? You have the power to spark change.

SIDE STORY:

There was a girl I knew who had to use left-over paper towels in her underwear for her period. Think about that… shocking, right? All of a sudden, you feel like you have it pretty good. Period poverty is a real problem in our communities. Reaching out and taking action is a way to make a real difference.

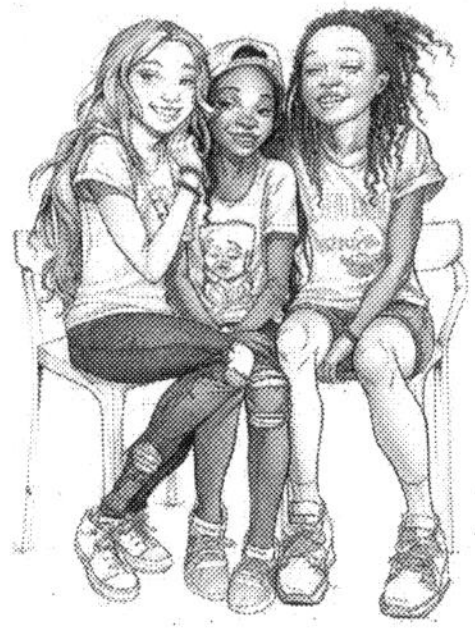

Wrapping Up: Your Period, Your Power

By now, you should feel like you've got a whole new perspective on your period. It's not just something to get through; it's a part of life that can actually bring some positives. It can bring a deeper understanding of your body, a chance to connect with others, and opportunities to fight for important causes.

Feeling empowered about your period takes time. Some days, you might be all about celebrating your cycle, and other days, it might still feel like a bit of a drag. That's totally okay. The important thing is that you're building a healthier, more positive relationship with your body and your period. It's based on knowledge, support, and yes, even a bit of fun.

I think it's really cool that you've arrived! Welcome, my friend!

Wear your period pride like a badge of honor! You've earned it! And who knows? You might inspire others to see their periods in a whole new light.

Your period is just one part of you, but it doesn't define you. You're way more powerful than any cramp, mood swing, or period mishap. By shifting how you view your period from a monthly thing that bugs you to a natural and manageable part of your life, you unlock a whole new level of confidence.

ACTION TAKEAWAYS:

- Continue to build your support squad.
- Create a fun party pack to welcome your period each month.
- Make fun plans during your period.
- Helping others less fortunate than you.
- Involve your parents in how you can find your period power. Use phrases like, "I'm on my period right now" to both of your parents, so that talking about periods is no big deal.

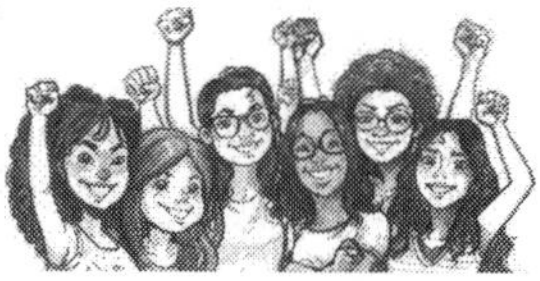

18. Around the World in 28 Days – The Period Edition

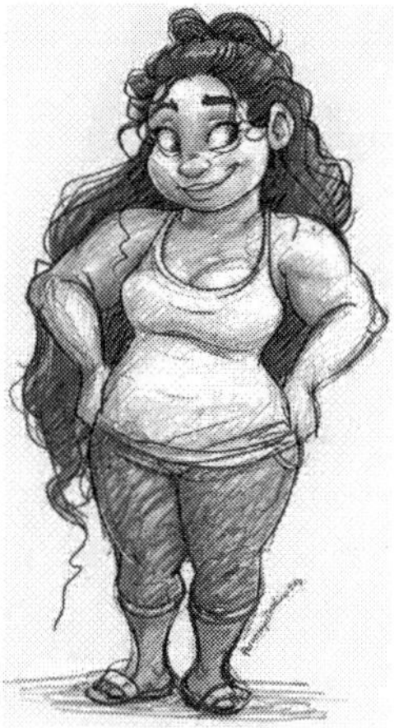

Hey, period adventurers! Are you ready to zoom around the globe and discover how girls, just like you, are rocking their period game in every corner of the planet? This is your all-access pass to discovering the wild, wonderful, and sometimes wacky world of menstruation across different cultures. It's like taking a world tour without leaving your room. And the ticket? Your period!

Let's Grab a Couple Facts

- Every month, around 26% of the people on this planet are having their menstrual cycle. Think about that! 26%! That means that if you look at four people in the market (or wherever), one of them will probably be on their period! Whaaaat?! This statistic is not based on every four women; this means out of every four PEOPLE! Yup, one out of every four people will be on their period!

- Additionally, that 26% means that 1.8 Billion (that's Billion—with a B!) people menstruate every month worldwide. Whoa! That's a lot of tampons, girl! Hahaha! But seriously, to let you know how big that number is, if you decided to count verbally to 1.8 Billion without stopping to sleep or eat 24 hours a day, it would take you about 172 years to count that high! That's HUGE!

Okay, now let's get back to you!

What's in the Period World Travel Kit?

If you're the one traveling, then of course you take all the period products that you know and love with you. Depending on where you land on this big ol' globe, the tools and gadgets you use for your period will be much different than you're used to as you travel around the world. It's like each place has its own period playlist.

- **Team Reusable:** In spots where being eco-friendly is the jam or where it's tough to get new pads every month, reusable pads are the stars of the show. They're old-school, but super cool.
- **The Menstrual Cup Revolution:** Picture this: A tiny cup that is saving the planet, one period at a time. From bustling cities in Europe to villages in the mountains of Nepal, menstrual cups are becoming the go-to for eco-savvy girls.
- **DIY Hacks:** In some corners of the world, period products are as rare as unicorn sightings. So, girls have become DIY experts, crafting their own pads from whatever's handy. It's all about that creative spirit.

Period Talk: From Taboo to Full-Blown Festivals

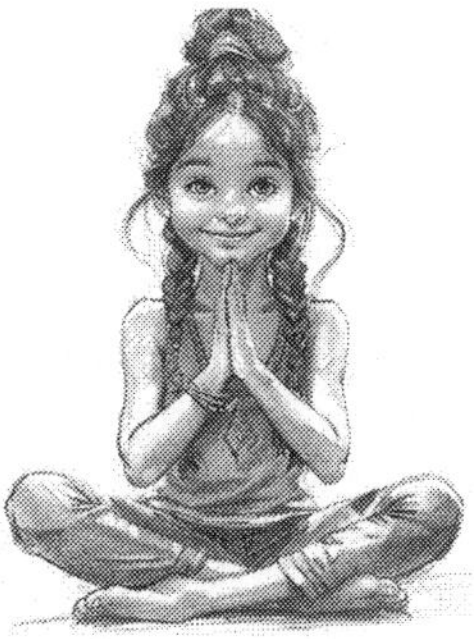

Let's chat about how periods are talked about (or not talked about) around the world.

- **Party Time in South India:** Yep, you've read that right. In Southern India, getting your first period is a big deal and calls for a celebration. They have a whole ceremony with gifts, feasts, and even fancy dresses. It's like a "Welcome to Womanhood" bash! Super Fun!
- **On the Flip Side, "Shhhh, it's a secret":** In some places, periods are super hush-hush, and you might not even talk about them with your friends. It's kind of like an unspoken rule that everyone follows. But slowly, things are starting to change as more people speak up. It seems weird to us, because we talk about things so openly, but that's not the case in other parts of the world.
- **School Struggles:** Imagine missing school because of your period. Sounds wild, right? But for some girls, that's a reality, especially if their schools don't have the right facilities or if period products are hard to come by.

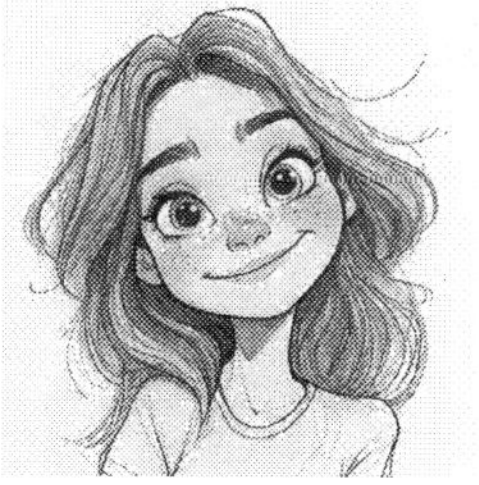

PERSONAL SIDE STORY:

Did you know that in some places, boys and girls learn together in class about puberty? I did. No joke. And it was embarrassing! I was squirming in my seat, trying not to look around, but then I noticed the boys were squirming, too. It was like this giant squirm-fest! Hahaha! But seriously, combined learning sort of normalizes the conversation from day one, so it's no biggie to chat about later.

The Period Posse: Global Edition

No matter where you are on the map, having a crew of supporters to help navigate the maze makes everything a bit easier.

- **Secret Handshakes (or Code Words):** From New York to Nairobi, girls have their own special signals for "I need a pad!" or "Period Emergency!" It's like being in an international spy network, but just for periods.
- **Digital Sisterhood:** Then there's the Internet, connecting period pals from all over the world with hashtags, memes, and stories. It's like having a BFF in every country, all united by your period experiences.
- **Breaking the Ice:** Even in cultures where talk is hush-hush, the ice is starting to crack. More and more girls are finding ways to support each other, through whispered conversations or shared online spaces.

The Grand Period Tour Wrap-Up

Whew! What a trip, right? Whether it's eco-friendly pads in Kenya, first-period parties in India, or secret signals shared between friends, it's clear we're all a part of a massive and amazing global period community.

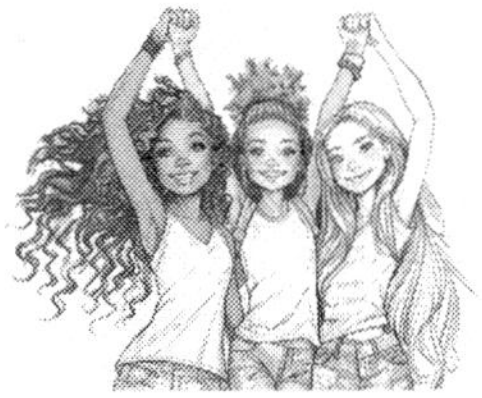

Next time you're dealing with cramps or racing to the bathroom to check for leaks, remember—you're part of a worldwide squad of incredible people navigating this journey. And each one of us, with our unique experiences and stories, is creating a beautiful mantra of period positivity that stretches across continents.

Keep exploring, keep sharing, and keep embracing your place in this global period posse! Because it doesn't matter where you are in the world, we're all riding the same menstrual cycle. You're just one member in a global string of connection, empowerment, and yes, a bit of adventure. All you have to do is reach out to the giant network. Here's to us, the worldwide wanderers of the period universe! Discovering new ideas and making waves, one cycle at a time.

Next up! How your period is your lifelong superpower!

ACTION TAKEAWAYS:

- Every month about 26% of the world is on its period.
- People in other countries use reusable pads, menstrual cups, or they come up with do-it-yourself kits in areas where supplies are not available.
- In some countries, getting your period can mean a huge party, but in other places, it means you can't even talk about it.
- Even though we live in different places around the world, we are all connected by this act of having a period. Kind of amazing!

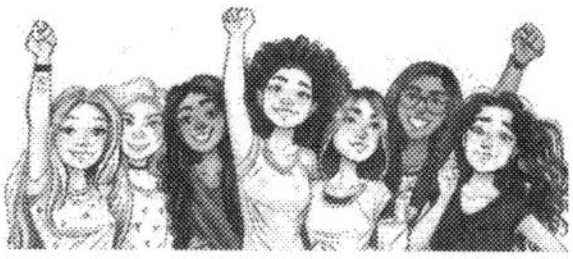

19. How Your Period Keeps You Sparkling Throughout Adulthood

Hey, Future Legends!

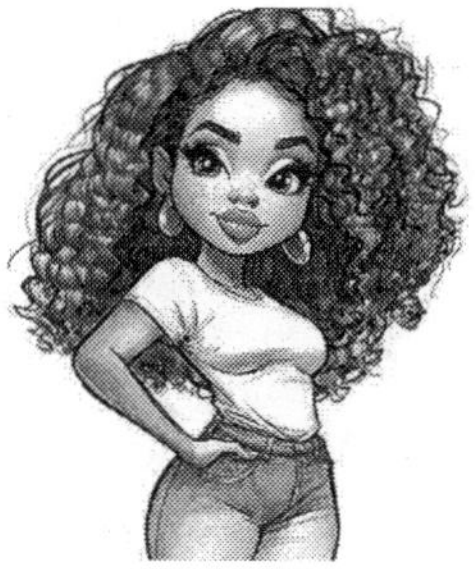

Since we've been going through this beautiful transition of periods together, you might be sitting there thinking to yourself: "Okay, so my period can be annoying, but seriously, what's the big picture?"

Well, get ready because I'm about to drop some truth bombs that will have you appreciating your period in a whole new way. And hear me out, they're the good kind of truth bombs—they're real breakthroughs!

There's a secret level we haven't fully explored yet. Your period isn't just a monthly visitor; it's more like your body's built-in upgrade, keeping you running at superhero status!

The Secret Sauce: Hormones!

First off, let's talk once again about these things called hormones. They're like the directors of your body's movie, telling different parts what to do and when. And guess what? The hormones that tag along with your period are actually your body's personal hocus-pocus magic.

- **Youth Potion!** You know how everyone's always searching for the secret to looking good and feeling young?—Bam!—your period hormones are part of that magic formula. They help your skin glow, your hair shine, and your overall vibe radiate confidence.
- **Bones of Steel!** Okay, maybe not steel, but your period hormones (especially estrogen) play a big role in keeping your bones strong. It's like they're your body's construction crew, making sure everything stays sturdy and ready for action.
- **Energizer Bunny Vibes!** Ever wonder why some days you feel like you can conquer the world? Yep, you guessed it, period hormones are at play again! They help regulate your energy levels to make sure you've got the juice to live your best life.

Growing Up: Your Period's Epic Journey

As you sail through the wild waves of tween life and into the open sea of teenhood, you one day finally arrive into the ocean of adulthood. And as you travel along, your period will carry you forward like your trusted BFF, growing and changing with you.

- **The Big Changes:** Just like you have changed from being a fan of hopscotch to mastering the sport of varsity basketball, your period is changing also. When it becomes more regular and you get better at predicting it, your period feels like less of a big deal.
- **The Deep Connection:** Your period isn't only about *bleeding* once a month; it's amazingly connected to how you feel, look, and even think. It's a sign that your body is doing all sorts of behind-the-scenes work to keep you at your best.

- **The Transformation:** Just like you upgrade from basic video games to the next level VR experiences, your period also levels up. You will become a period-navigating ninja, dodging cramps like a boss, knowing exactly what your body needs.

The Ultimate Achievement: Period Positivity

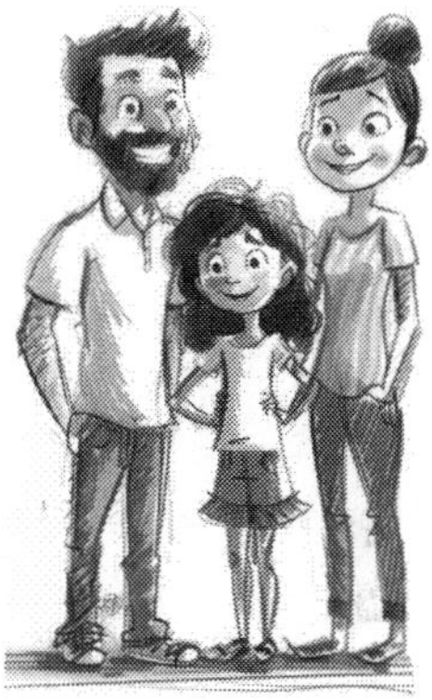

Okay awesome humans, as we wrap up this chapter, I hope you're feeling a newfound respect and maybe even a bit of love for your period. Sure, it can be kind of a pain sometimes, but it's also your body's way of keeping you youthful, sparkling, strong, and full of energy.

Keep rocking, keep learning, and remember: Your period is more than just a monthly event; it's a key player in the amazing journey of being you. So, here's to embracing that journey—hormones, periods, and all—because they're all part of what makes you uniquely fabulous now and into your future!

ACTION TAKEAWAYS:

- Hormones are the "secret sauce" that keeps you looking young, strong, and beautiful throughout your adulthood.
- Your hormones create an environment where you can have deeper and more adult thoughts. You will start to have opinions on things that you feel matter, and you will feel a deep connection to the world.

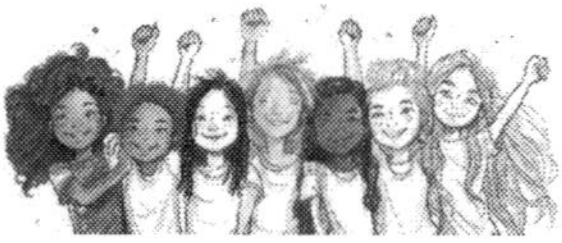

20. Doc Talk and Beyond

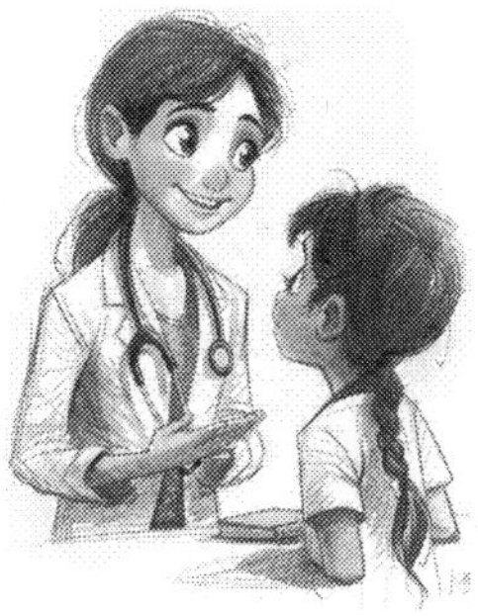

Hey there, superstar! We've had an incredible journey together, right? From figuring out the mysteries of mood swings to handling the pain for period cramps—we've grown, and maybe even had a few "Aha!" moments along the way. We're down to where we have one of our last chats, and it's super important.

The Ultimate Health Advisors: Your Doctors

As much fun as we've had spilling the beans on all things period-related, there's something super crucial you've got to remember: This book, as awesome as it is, doesn't replace your doctor or any medical pro. I know, I know, I'm fun, and your doctors might seem like they speak another language, but they're on your team. They're like the ultimate co-operative partner in the game of health.

Think of your doctor as your personal health superhero. They've got this superpower of medical knowledge that can seem like magic, but it's actually science. Cool, right? Here's why they rock and deserve their own special theme music:

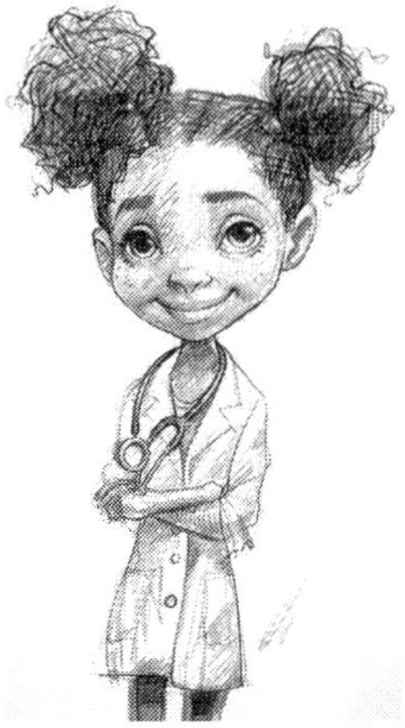

- **Brainy Bunch:** They know stuff—A LOT of stuff. Your doctor spent a gazillion years in school just so they can help you out. They know the ins, the outs, the ups, and the downs of bodies just like yours. So when they give advice, it's worth a listen.
- **Custom Power-Ups:** Just like you choose power-ups in video games based on the level you're tackling, doctors can give you medical power-ups made only for you. It's like having a secret weapon against period problems.
- **Personalized Game Plan:** While this book gives you a general overview, your doc can provide a game plan made just for you.
- **Confidence Crew:** Worried about sharing personal stuff? Docs are like vaults, trained to keep your secrets locked up tighter than a diary. They're all about making sure you feel safe and heard.

When to Hit Up Your Doctor

Not sure when to make that appointment? Here are some prime times to check in:

- **Cramp-zilla!** If cramps are making you wish for an alien abduction, it's time to see your doctor. They can help make sure everything's okay and suggest ways to lessen the pain.
- **Mood Swings on Steroids?** Feeling a bit more emotional than what you think is normal—like you're riding a mega

rollercoaster of feelings? Your doctor can help level things out.

- **Flow Like Whoa?** Is your period so heavy, you're thinking of investing in a rubber raft? Definitely talk to your doctor. They can check for any underlying causes and help you find solutions.

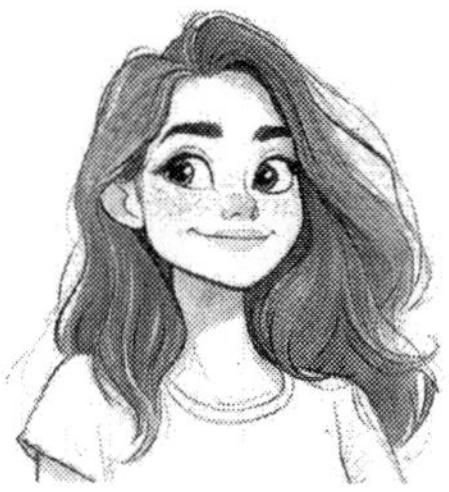

BONUS PRO TIP:

Make a list of your issues and extra needs. Lists help remind us of all the important things we need to do or say. Once you start using lists, you'll probably never stop. Have your list include what you're having a difficult time with (and why), plus any unusual entries in your ***MY PERIOD POWER! WORKBOOK.***

Bring your list and workbook to help you remember what to bring up during your visit. We sometimes get excited and forget what to tell our doctors, so a list comes in really handy. Since doctors are only able to spend a short amount of time with us, we need to be efficient with their time. (FYI, I make lists and take them when I go into the doctor, also!)

Bringing your notes in will help the doctor see if and when there is a repeating issue. Sometimes, it's good to tell your doctor, "Hey, every month ___________ happens." Talking it out is how we can make things better!

Real Talk: Real Doctors vs. Dr. Internet

Here we are, nearing the end of our epic quest. You're now armed with knowledge, empowered to take on your period like a boss, and ready to live your best life every day of the month.

Part of being a boss is knowing when to call in the experts, which means your friendly neighborhood doctor. Even though we have the world wide web at our fingertips, an internet search does not arm you with *specific* information for *your* specific needs. It only gives you *general* information about the *average* of the *world's* needs. See the difference? A doctor's advice is tailored only for you. Also, keep in mind that internet advice is only as good as what you paid for it, which is usually nothing. Plus, some results you get on an internet search can be terrifying! Go to the experts. Go see your personal doctor!

And never forget: Your health is your superpower! Use it, protect it, and when in doubt, ask the pros.

Next, probably THE MOST IMPORTANT CHAPTER IN THE BOOK... Drumroll, please!!

ACTION TAKEAWAYS:

- Analyze: "Do I need to talk to my doctor?" Include your parents in this discussion.
- Write down symptoms, special issues, and other important items that you need to discuss with your doctor. You can even write them down in your ***MY PERIOD POWER! WORKBOOK!***
- The Internet is no substitute for a real doctor's advice.

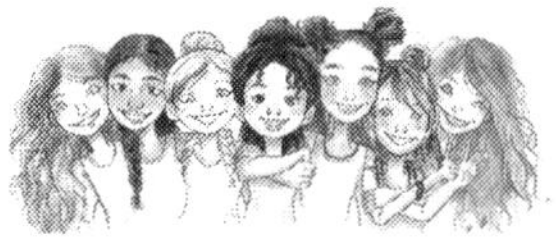

21. Last Chapter: THE MOST IMPORTANT CHAPTER In This Book!

Superhero Action—All Month Long, All Year Long, All Life Long!

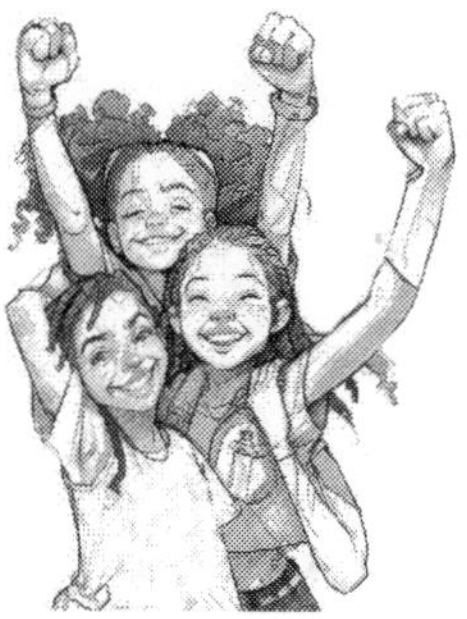

Hey you, Superstar! Can you believe that we're already at the end of the book? Congratulate yourself on your own personal growth!

I know we've been focusing a ton on what happens when we're actually on our period. Some of it takes getting used to, but here's the scoop: The rest of the month is just as important for keeping your vibe high and yourself feeling awesome, for like, forever!

Let's break down why taking care of yourself, even when you're not *"during that time of the month,"* is your secret sauce to rocking your period power all month long, all year long, all life long.

Who Do You Want To Be When You Grow Older?

Treat yourself and reach for those wild dreams! Go on, you can do it! I'd love to hear all about your success stories!

I ask this now, not because you need to know exactly *WHAT* you want to be when you grow older, but because it is important to start figuring out *WHO* you want to be and create that positive mental attitude. You may not know it, but your adult life has now begun!

Congratulations and Welcome to the Big Show!

Belief in yourself and your skills is a huge part of getting where you want to be in life. What a great time to learn this! While you're adapting yourself to understanding your body, you might as well apply these same ideas to build great life skills.

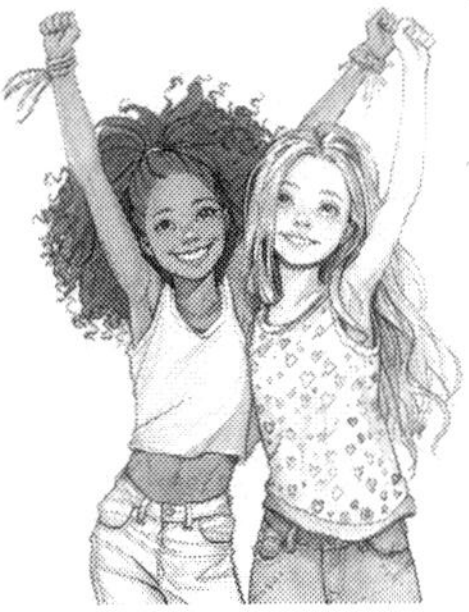

This May Be the Most Important Part of This Book (And I'm Not Kidding!)

Hidden within these chapters, where I've been writing (and joking around) about dealing with your periods, mastering your mood swings, and taking care of your body, these are literally the same skills you need to master the skill of life!! Whaaaaat?! Yeah, that's right!

You have all the basic tools in your toolbox now, so rework some of these sentences, wiggle the word "period" out of "My Period Power!" and guess what you're left with—**"MY POWER!"**

That's right! Say it out loud! "MY POWER!!" Scream it, if you want! "MY POWER!!"

Hahahaha!! I love it! Because, you know what? You can own this, this power of yours. And trust me, I'm not joking with you—when you believe it and you live it, YOU LITERALLY ARE POWERFUL!

So say, "Take that, you crummy period-dog, you puberty monster! You're not going to get the best of me! I've got MY POWER! I've got all these great tools to slay you and any other fire-breathing dragon that comes along my path!"

Because having this period every month:

- Is making me stronger!
- Is making me wiser!
- Is making me take care of myself!
- Is making me understand that all the strength that lies within me is only just starting to wake up!

Exciting, isn't it?!

Who knew that getting your period was going to be so outrageously important?

Every woman who has walked before you has had her period, <u>but not every woman has understood her power.</u>

I think I should repeat that, because it is so important!—**<u>not every woman has understood her power.</u>**

Please take this beautiful change in your life, and instead of just getting through it, instead of letting it rule you, take your amazing power and own it! Go forth and conquer it, warrior queen!

<u>IMPORTANT:</u> Yes, all of these ideas are great, but you have to apply them to your life to make them work.

I repeat, **YOU HAVE TO APPLY THESE IDEAS TO YOUR LIFE TO MAKE THEM WORK!**

Now Let's Switch Our Talk to YOU, Who Now Owns All of this Incredible Knowledge!

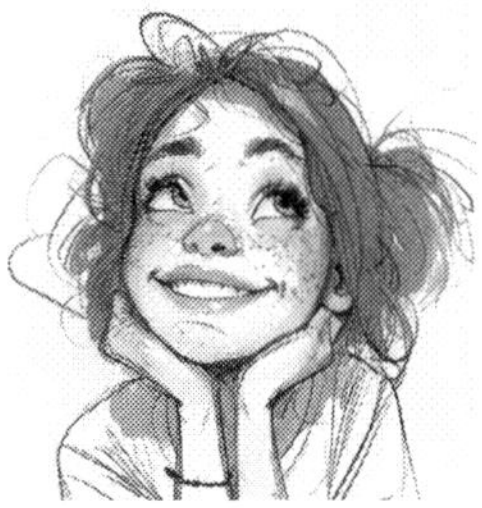

I NOW KNOW HOW TO:

1. Track my cycle!
2. Monitor my moods!
3. Keep track of my water intake!
4. Enjoy a healthy diet!
5. Crush those Cramps!
6. Use my period gear!
7. Take care of my grooming!
8. Keep an eye on my sleep needs!
9. Track my supplies!
10. Appreciate my friends!
11. Keep my attitude positive!
12. Educate others!
13. Not keep my tampon in more than 4-6 hours, MAX!
14. Be a support to others!
15. Deal with my pain!
16. Listen to my body!
17. Deal with my emotions!
18. Laugh instead of cry!
19. Say NO to things that aren't right for me!
20. Seek out reliable advice!
21. Think and talk about myself in a positive way!
22. Know that I'm not alone!
23. Talk with my parents or a trusted adult to find the answers to my questions, or to vent my feelings!
24. Have good people that I look up to!
25. Cut myself some slack!
26. Deal with guys!
27. Embrace my body!
28. Prepare for my future self!

29. And… **<u>FEEL MY POWER!</u>**

My period is just the first step in this beautiful dream we call life. And I understand that what was once "My Period Power!" is now actually me claiming my strength, my body, "<u>MY POWER!</u>"

♥♥♥

Thank you for letting *<u>MY PERIOD POWER!</u>* be a part of this journey with you! I hope you found this book helpful.

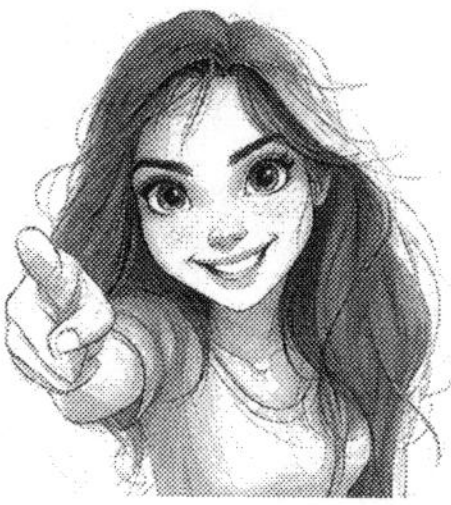

Help someone else find the help they need! You can be the reason for their success!

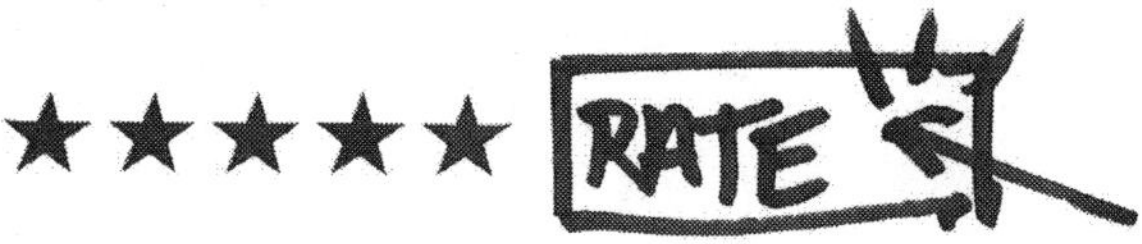

1. Use the link or QR code:

https://dub.sh/APPA

2. <u>Share your feelings</u>: How did it help you? Did it make you smile? Did you have an "Oh, I get it now!" moment?

3. Please leave a <u>GREAT STARS</u> ★★★★★ <u>WRITTEN REVIEW</u> letting everyone know what you loved about the book, so other people will get the help they need also!

4. <u>Maybe add a picture or video</u> of yourself along with your review and online talking about how the book helped you! I'd love to see who you are! **#MyPeriodPower!**

Want more tools for your confidence journey? Check out these other empowering reads:

- ***MY SOCIAL POWER!*** (For Boy & Girl Tweens, Teens, and Young Adults)
- ***MY BODY POWER!*** (For Girl Tweens, Teens, and Young Adults)
- ***MY SOCIAL POWER! WORKBOOK*** (For Boy & Girl Tweens, Teens, and Young Adults)
- ***MY PERIOD POWER! WORKBOOK*** (For Girl Tweens, Teens, and Young Adults)

They are the perfect companions for your puberty journey.

THANK YOU!
Now go out and grab your POWER!

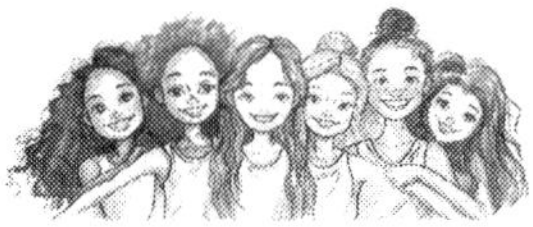

Acknowledgements

Writing ***MY PERIOD POWER!*** has been such an incredible experience, and it would not have been possible without the love and support of so many amazing people who helped me along the way.

First and foremost, a huge thank you to YOU—the reader! Whether you're just starting out on your journey with body confidence or you've been building body confidence for a while, I'm so proud of you for picking up this book. I wrote it with you in mind, and I hope it gives you the tools you need to feel strong, empowered, and confident in your own skin. I'm so excited to be a part of your journey! You're amazing, just as you are.

A big thank you to my incredible family, who have always encouraged me to be bold and go after my dreams. You've given me the confidence to pursue projects like this one, and your endless love and support mean the world to me. To my incredible family—especially my parents —for always encouraging me to dream big and never give up on my big dreams. You taught me the importance of self-love and confidence, and that has shaped everything I have done in my life and have written.

I also want to express my deepest gratitude to Dr. Renee Cotter, who graciously wrote the foreword for ***MY PERIOD POWER!*** Your expertise, wisdom, and passion for helping young people embrace their bodies have had a huge impact on me and this book. While you didn't write this book, your support and guidance have been invaluable, and I'm so thankful to have your voice included.

To all the health professionals, educators, and body positivity advocates out there: Thank you for the important work you do every day. Your efforts to empower young people to love themselves and to take care of their bodies inspire me, and this book wouldn't be what it is without the important work you've contributed to this field.

Lastly, a massive shout-out to my talented publishing team who brought ***MY PERIOD POWER!*** to life. Every detail of this book has your magic touch, and I'm so grateful for your dedication and hard work in making this project shine.

To every young person reading this—thank you for being brave, curious, and open to learning more about your body. I hope this book helps you embrace the changes, challenges, and joys that come with growing up.

A Special Note to You, the Reader…

You are powerful and wonderful, and I believe in you every step of the way.

With love and gratitude,

SheriBelle Karper

About the Author

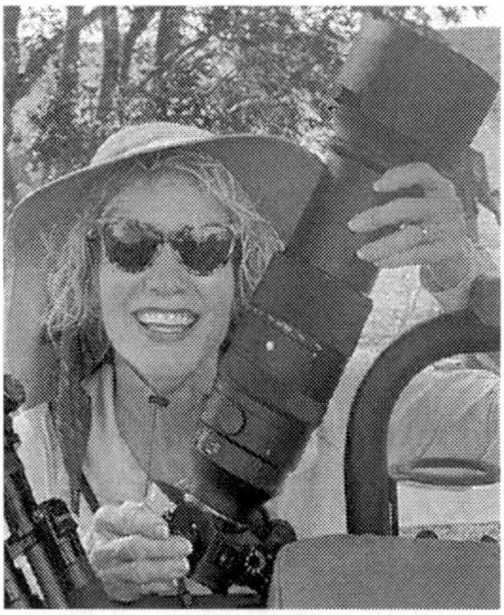

SheriBelle Karper is a true citizen of the world, uniquely equipped to share wisdom on confidence and self-empowerment. For years, she's been an adventure photographer, traveling across the globe (often solo), seeking out new faces, wild places, and unforgettable experiences. She has set foot in a jaw-dropping number of countries. That kind of globetrotting takes some serious confidence.

Through all her travels, SheriBelle has had a front-row seat to some of life's most extraordinary moments. She's danced with tribes in Africa, petted wild Icelandic ponies, and whacked her way through the dense jungles of northern Thailand while trekking alongside elephants. She stood among the solemn bomb sites of Sarajevo, witnessing history's lingering scars, and watched families in Nepal say sacred goodbyes during beautiful afterlife ceremonies. From joy to loss, from wilderness to wonder—she's seen it all.

One of her most unforgettable moments? When she traveled solo to the country of Tonga to freedive in the vast Tongan Trench! (It is the second-deepest ocean trench on Earth, plunging more than an astonishing 35,000 feet. Although, she didn't freedive that far down!) Swimming in those wild, rolling waters—only a few yards from massive humpback whale mothers and their newborn calves—she captured the magic through her professional underwater camera lens. SheriBelle recalls locking eyes with one mother whale, describing it like this: "It felt like I was right there with something god-like, something beyond words, something immensely powerful—like whatever created the sun and the moon… That kind of power? That kind of connection? That kind of adventure? Yep, that takes confidence!

In 2018, when Hawaii's Big Island was first rocked by a volcanic eruption, SheriBelle Karper was right there, capturing history in real time. She spent five intense days behind the lines with the National Guard, shooting alongside media giants like CNN, Fox News, and NBC. Only a few crews were allowed to go back each day, and SheriBelle was among them. Wearing a hardhat, goggles, and a gas mask, she listened as the National Guard's monitors beeped louder and faster—warning of deadly gases in the air. At one point, the wind shifted. She and the team had to sprint to safety, their vans screeching away, just in time. She even took three daring open-door helicopter flights to photograph the lava spewing beneath her. Sitting up front with the pilot, leaning halfway out of the chopper with her camera in hand, SheriBelle captured the breathtaking chaos of that erupting volcano. Fearless confidence, indeed!

But SheriBelle's boldness isn't confined to her global adventures. She's also a multi-award-winning and nominated screenwriter and author, celebrated for her comedic wit and sharp storytelling. She's even taken the mic at Los Angeles's legendary comedy club, *The Improv*, performing stand-up for live audiences. Stand-up comedy? That's another arena where confidence is a must!

Her social impact extends beyond the wild and the far away. At home, SheriBelle has spent years empowering young people. She served on the board of a major charity supporting at-risk youth, spearheaded a graffiti-removal program in partnership with a major paint company, and even trained in grief counseling for high school students because she believes so deeply in helping teens navigate life's tough moments.

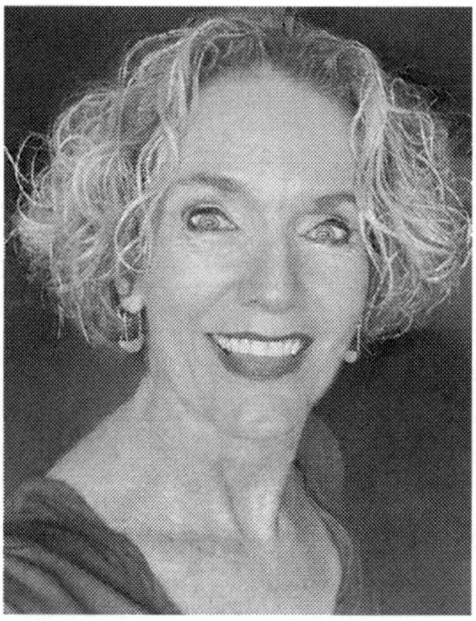

She's been acknowledged by Los Angeles City and County leaders for her dedication to creating opportunities for teens. She's even enjoyed many years of volunteering at her kids' schools, where she's seen first-hand how confidence and curiosity go hand-in-hand.

And while all of SheriBelle's adventures are extraordinary, her greatest and most fulfilling experience has been raising her two children—her ultimate source of pride. In her words, "They are beautiful and gifted in each their own way, and live fearlessly, with humor and honor." While raising them, SheriBelle has practiced everything she shares in her books, proof that confidence begins at home.

SheriBelle has had all these extraordinary life experiences: From photographing the world's wildest corners to free-diving with whales, to cracking jokes on world-famous stages, to winning awards for her writing, to raising two amazing kids, to fleeing a violent volcano, just to name a few. And somehow, still made it back in time for school pickup. All of these experiences have shaped SheriBelle Karper into a woman who knows what it takes to face life's challenges head-on. She knows that she can trust herself and move through the world with strength and courage. Now, she's bringing that same bold spirit to her writing, crafting confidence guides like ***MY SOCIAL POWER!, MY BODY POWER!, MY PERIOD POWER!, MY SOCIAL POWER! WORKBOOK,*** and ***MY PERIOD POWER! WORKBOOK,*** to help young people discover their own inner power and confidence during this very important time of their lives.

Whether she's swimming with humpbacks, writing award-winning stories, or helping teens embrace their unique journeys, SheriBelle

Karper is on a mission to inspire confidence in all its forms, and she's here to help *you* find yours!

Now it's your turn! What will your adventure be? What kind of confidence are you ready to grow? Whether it's making a new friend, trying something new, or speaking up for what matters to you. This is your moment. Let's go!

Other Titles by SheriBelle Karper

— —YOUNG ADULT— —

<u>The MY POWER! Series</u>
https://Dub.sh/MyPowerSeries

MY BODY POWER! (Body Confidence Guide: For Girls - Tweens, Teens and Young Adults) ★★★★★

https://Dub.sh/MyBodyPowerBook
Also Available In Spanish. Soon in French, German, Italian, European Portuguese, Brazilian Portuguese, Japanese, Simplified Chinese, and Russian

MY SOCIAL POWER! (Social Confidence Guide: For Boys & Girls - Tweens, Teens and Young Adults) ★★★★★

https://Dub.sh/MySocialPowerBook
Also Available In Spanish. Soon in French, German, Italian, European

Portuguese, Brazilian Portuguese, Japanese, Simplified Chinese, and Russian

MY PERIOD POWER! WORKBOOK (Period Confidence Workbook: For Girls - Tweens, Teens and Young Adults) ★★★★★

Also Available In Spanish. Soon in French, German, Italian, European Portuguese, Brazilian Portuguese, Japanese, Simplified Chinese, and Russian

MY SOCIAL POWER! WORKBOOK (Social Confidence Workbook: For Boys & Girls - Tweens, Teens and Young Adults) ★★★★★

Also Available In Spanish. Soon in French, German, Italian, European Portuguese, Brazilian Portuguese, Japanese, Simplified Chinese, and Russian

— —MEMOIR— —

WHY THE WIDOW WEARS BLACK ★★★★★

Please check out all the other titles at KingmanPublications.com

Kingman Publications LLC

Glossary and Words to Know!

Acceptance: Being cool with who you are and where you are in life. It's not about trying to change everything about yourself, but embracing your awesome one-of-a-kind self.

Acetaminophen: It's a kind of medicine you can take when you have a headache or cramps during your period. It helps make the pain chill out. Make sure that you **talk to your parents and your doctor prior to taking any medication.**

Acne: When your skin gets all bumpy and red, because of too much oil, dead skin, and dirt clogging your pores. It's like your skin's way of saying it needs a good wash!

Amenorrhea: This is when someone doesn't get their period for a while. It's not about having it once, and then skipping; it's more like never starting or taking a very long break. Could be because of stress, diet, or too much exercise.

Areolae: The dark circles around your nipples, kind of like a bull's-eye, but for where babies feed.

Attributes: The cool qualities and characteristics that make you unique, like being funny, kind, or creative. Your attributes are what make you YOU!

Authentic: Being 100% real and true to who you are. No faking or pretending; just being you.

Beauty Standards: What people think is "beautiful" based on what they see in the media or around them. These standards change all the time, so don't let them define you.

Birth Control: These are the ways to stop you from getting pregnant when you're older and decide to be physically intimate with someone. There are lots of types, like pills, or special devices a doctor can help with. This is not really a subject that we will cover in this book, but it is a very important subject to discuss with your parents and doctor.

Blackheads: Dark spots on your skin, especially your nose and forehead, where oil, dead skin, and dirt have gotten stuck and turned dark.

Bloating: Ever feel like your belly is all puffy and full of air? That's bloating. It can happen before or during your period, and makes your clothes feel tighter.

Body Confidence: Feeling awesome about your body and loving it for what it is, no matter the size, shape, or what anyone else says.

Body Image: How you see and feel about your body, which can change based on your mood or what's going on around you.

Body Positivity: The belief that all bodies are beautiful, no matter the shape or size. It's about loving your body for what it is by talking and thinking about it positively.

Body Shaming: When someone makes mean comments about another person's body. It's totally not OK and says more about them than you.

Boundaries: The personal limits you set to protect your feelings, space, and time. They help you feel safe and respected, and saying "no" is totally OK.

Breast Bud: The early bump under your nipple that shows your breasts are starting to grow. It's the first step in getting boobs!

Bullying: When someone is mean on purpose, whether it's online or in real life. It's not cool, and it's never your fault. Don't be afraid to speak up!

Caffeine: A zippy ingredient in coffee and soda that can keep you awake and bouncing off the walls if you have too much. It isn't good to have it too late in the day. Rest is very important during your period.

Calcium: Super important mineral for your bones, making them strong and tough. It creates a sturdy skeleton.

Clitoris: A tiny, sensitive spot at the top of your vulva.

Comparison: When you look at someone else and start thinking their life or body is better than yours. Don't fall for it—you're one of a kind!

Compassion: Being kind and understanding toward others and yourself, especially when someone's going through a tough time.

Confidence: Walking into a room, knowing you're amazing. It's like giving yourself a high five every day.

Consent: A big deal word that means saying yes or no to things that affect your body. It's about making sure everyone's cool with what's happening.

Cramps: Ouch! These are the achy pains in your lower belly you get when your period shows up. It's like your body's way of telling you it's cleaning house.

Criticism: When someone points out what they think is wrong about something you do or how you look. It can be helpful or harmful, but it doesn't define you.

Cycle Tracking: Keeping an eye on when your period comes and goes, so you can guess when it'll visit next. Helps to not get surprised by your period's "hello," and doesn't catch you off guard.

Dandruff: Annoying white flakes in your hair, coming from your scalp. It's like your head's way of saying it needs some extra tender, loving care (TLC!).

Delayed Puberty: When your body takes a bit longer to start the growing and changing phase.

Dermatologist: A doctor who knows all about skin and helps you when you have pimples, rashes, or other skin stuff going on.

Diet Culture: All those messages telling you to lose weight or change your body to fit some "ideal." Heads up: you don't need to change anything about yourself to be beautiful!

Discharge: A gooey, slimy stuff (sometimes whitish) that comes out of your vagina. It is totally natural and part of your body keeping itself clean.

Diversity: Celebrating what makes everyone unique, like different looks, cultures, and backgrounds. Because being different is what makes life cool!

Dysmenorrhea: A fancy word for super painful cramps. Like, when the cramps are so bad, you just want to curl up in a ball and not move.

Empowerment: That powerful feeling when you know you can do anything. It's like having your own personal superpower!

Empathy: Understanding how someone else feels, like putting yourself in their shoes. It's what makes you a kind and caring friend.

Endometrium: It's the inside layer of your uterus that build up every month to get ready for a baby. If there's no baby, it breaks down and comes out as your period.

Estrogen: One of the body's hormones that helps girls become women, especially during puberty. It also plays a big part in the menstrual cycle.

Exercise: Moving your body in a way that makes you feel good. It could be dancing, running, swimming, or anything that gets you active.

Fallopian Tubes: The twisty pathways in your body, where eggs travel from your ovaries to your womb, like nature's little conveyor belts.

Fertility: It's about whether you can make a baby. When you're older, fertility means your body is ready to get pregnant if you decide to have kids.

FSH: This stands for Follicle-Stimulating Hormone. It's a hormone that tells your ovaries to get an egg ready each month for your period cycle.

FOMO: It stands for Fear Of Missing Out. That feeling when you think everyone's having fun without you. But remember, you're not missing out on being awesome!

Genitals: Your private parts down there, including your vulva, vagina, and everything inside and out that's involved in the reproductive system.

Goals: Things you want to achieve, like acing a test or learning a new skill. Setting goals helps you grow and become even more amazing!

Gratitude: Focusing on the things you're thankful for, like your friends, your health, or even your favorite snack. It can only help you feel happier!

Growing Pains: The aches and pains you feel in your body, especially legs, as you stretch and grow taller during growth spurts.

Growth Spurt: When you suddenly grow a lot taller in a short time, like you're shooting up faster than a weed in the garden.

Gynecologist: The doctor that you go to for female-related health and problems. They are your go-to source for all period matters. You will continue to see your gynecologist throughout your adult health journey.

Healthy Eating: Eating a variety of foods that give you energy and make your body feel good. It's about balance, not perfection.

Healthy Habits: The little things you do every day, like drinking water, eating good food, and moving your body, to feel your best inside and out.

Hormones: These are like your body's messengers. They tell different parts of your body what to do, like when to grow, or when it's time for your period.

Hygiene: This is about keeping clean, especially during your period. It means changing pads or tampons regularly and washing up to feel and smell fresh.

Inclusivity: Making sure everyone feels welcome and accepted, no matter who they are, what they look like, or where they come from.

Inner Beauty: What makes you beautiful on the inside: things like kindness, confidence, and being a good friend. That's the stuff that really shines!

Inner Critic: That little voice in your head that sometimes says negative things about you. It's important to challenge it and not let it bring you down.

Insecurity: That icky feeling when you're unsure about yourself or how you look. Spoiler: everyone feels this sometimes, but it's OK—you're awesome just as you are!

Insomnia: When sleep plays hard to get, and you can't fall asleep, or stay asleep, no matter how tired you are.

Intercourse: A grown-up thing where two people's bodies come together in a special, intimate way, often relating to making babies.

Ibuprofen: A medicine that helps with pain and swelling. Great for tackling those period cramps or when you've got a headache. Make sure you talk to your parents and doctor prior to taking any medication.

Journaling: Writing down your thoughts, feelings, or experiences to help you understand yourself better and work through emotions.

Labia: The two sets of "lips" around your vaginal opening, part of the vulva, that help protect and cover your inner private parts.

LH Surge: This stands for Luteinizing Hormone Surge. It's a big hormone wave that tells an egg to leave the ovary. It's a key part of the menstrual cycle.

Media: TV shows, social media, magazines, and everything you watch or read. Sometimes it's awesome, but not everything you see is real life.

Meditation: Chilling out on purpose. Sitting quietly and letting your mind take a break from all the noise and busyness.

Menarche: Fancy term for your first ever period. It's a big step in becoming a teenager and means your body is doing its thing.

Menopause: Way later in life, when a woman's period says "bye-bye" for good, and she stops being able to have babies.

Mental Health: How you're feeling in your brain and your heart, like whether you're happy, stressed, or anxious. Just like your body, your mind needs care, too.

Menstrual Cup: A reusable cup you can use instead of pads or tampons. It catches your period blood and is eco-friendly because you wash and reuse it.

Menstrual Cycle: The whole process your body goes through to get ready for a possible baby each month, ending with your period if there's no baby.

Menstrual Equity: This is about making sure everyone who gets their period has what they need, like pads or tampons, no matter their money situation.

Menstrual Hygiene: All about taking care of yourself during your period using period products the right way and keeping clean to stay comfy and healthy.

Menstrual Phase: This part of your menstrual cycle is when you actually have your period. It's the body's way of getting rid of the inner lining of the uterus when there's no baby.

Menstrual Products: These are items like pads, tampons, and menstrual cups that you use to manage your period. They help collect the blood so you can go about your day.

Menstruation: Another name for your period. It's when blood and tissue from your uterus come out through your vagina. It's a normal part of being a girl and happens once a month.

Mindfulness: Paying attention to what's happening right now, like how you're feeling or breathing, without getting stressed about it. It's not about thinking about the past or the future, it's only the RIGHT NOW.

Mindset: The way you think about yourself and the world around you. A positive outlook can help you achieve your goals.

Mood Swings: When your feelings change super fast, like being happy one minute and sad the next. It can happen around your period because of hormone changes.

Negative Self-Talk: Those not-so-nice thoughts about yourself that pop-up sometimes. The key is learning to flip them into positive self-talk.

Nipples: The pointy bit on your breast where milk comes out if you ever have a baby. They can be sensitive to the touch.

NSAIDs: These are nonsteroidal anti-inflammatory drugs. These are medicines like ibuprofen that help with pain and swelling. Good for dealing with cramps. Make sure you talk to your doctor and parents prior to taking any medication.

Ova: A fancy word for eggs, the ones in your ovaries, not the fridge! They're part of what can make a baby when the time is right.

Ovaries: These are two small organs that hold all your eggs. They also make hormones like estrogen and progesterone, which help control your period.

Ovulation: This is part of your menstrual cycle, when an ovary releases an egg. It's the time when you can get pregnant if you're older and having sexual intercourse.

Pads: Pads are like soft, absorbent stickers you put in your underwear to catch blood. They come in different sizes for light or heavy days.

Peer Pressure: When friends or classmates try to nudge you into doing something you're not so sure about. It's like the pushy friend that tries to convince you to do something that you may not want to do. It is very important to talk to your parents, or a trusted adult, if someone is pressuring you to do something you don't feel is right for you.

Pelvic Inflammatory Disease (PID): This is an infection in the female reproductive organs. It's not about your period. It can be caused by STDs so it's important to know about for your health.

Perfectionism: When you think you have to do everything 100% right all the time. Spoiler alert: Nobody's perfect, and that's OK. Don't worry about perfection, because it's impossible.

Period: Another word for menstruation. It's the few days each month when blood comes out of your vagina, a sign that your body is working right.

Period Poverty: This is when girls and women can't afford period products, which makes it hard for them to go to school or work during their period.

Period Stigma: This is a weird or negative attitude some people have about periods. It's not cool, because menstruation is natural and happens to half of the population.

Period Tracking: Your ***MY PERIOD POWER! WORKBOOK***, and other tools like this that can help you keep track of your menstrual cycle. It can help you predict when your period will start and help you notice any patterns or changes.

Period Underwear: Special underwear that has extra layers to absorb your period blood. You can wear them instead of, or as a backup to pads or tampons.

Polycystic Ovary Syndrome (PCOS): A health condition where women have higher levels of certain hormones, which can make periods irregular and cause other symptoms like hair growth and acne.

PMS (Pre-Menstrual Syndrome): The physical and emotional symptoms that some girls and women get before their period starts, like cramps, mood swings, and bloating.

Positive Affirmations: Little pep talks you give yourself, like "I am strong" or "I love my body." Saying them out loud or in your head can seriously boost your mood.

Positivity: Focusing on the good stuff in life, like the things you love about yourself, instead of what you don't.

Precocious Puberty: When puberty shows up, super early, like a guest arriving way before the party starts.

Progesterone: A hormone your body makes that helps control your menstrual cycle and gets your uterus ready for a possible pregnancy each month.

Puberty: The big change-o-rama, when your body goes from kid to teen, getting ready for all the grown-up stuff, like growing hair and new places, getting taller, and starting your periods.

Reflection: Taking time to think about your thoughts, feelings, or what's going on in your life. It helps you understand yourself better and make better choices.

Reproductive Health: This is all about the health of your reproductive system. It includes periods, but also things like going to the gynecologist and making sure everything is working right.

Resilience: The ability to bounce back when things get tough. It's like having an inner strength that helps keep you going, even when stuff gets hard.

Role Models: People you look up to because they inspire you. They can be anyone from celebrities to your BFF, as long as they help you reach for how awesome you can be.

Sanitary Napkins: Another name for pads. They're used to absorb period blood and keep you feeling clean and dry.

Self-Esteem: How you feel about yourself, like how much you think you're amazing. (by the way, you totally are!)

Self-Expression: Showing the world who you are through your style, hobbies, or the things you say and do. It's how you let your unique personality shine.

Self-Image: How you picture yourself in your head. Sometimes it's good, sometimes not-so-good, but it's all about learning to love what you see.

Self-Love: Treating yourself with kindness and respect, like you would your best friend. It's about being your own biggest fan.

Self-Talk: The things you say to yourself in your head. Positive self-talk can make you feel strong, negative self-talk can bring you down. Choose kindness!

Self-Worth: Knowing that you're valuable and amazing no matter what anyone else says.

Sexual Health: This is about taking care of your reproductive system, and making safe choices about sex. It includes using protection and getting checked for sexually transmitted diseases and infections.

Sexual Intercourse: When two adults get really close and connect their bodies in a way they can show love or make babies. It's part of grown-up relationships.

Social Media: Apps like Instagram, TikTok, Facebook or Snapchat, where people post photos and videos. It can be fun, but what you see isn't always real life.

Spotting: This is light bleeding that can happen between periods, or when you're not expecting your period. It's usually nothing to worry about, but can be a sign to check in with a doctor if it keeps happening.

Stretch Marks: Little lines that show up on your skin when you grow fast. Totally normal, and a sign that your body is changing—no biggie!

Support System: The people who've got your back, like friends, family, or teachers. They're there to lift you up when you need it most.

Sustainable Menstruation: Using products like menstrual cups, reusable pads, or period underwear to help the environment. It's all about having a period without creating a lot of trash.

Tampons: A product you insert into your vagina to absorb blood. They come in different sizes for different flow levels and are invisible from the outside.

Toxic: When someone or something is super negative and brings you down. Whether it's a person or a situation, you don't need that bad energy in your life.

Toxic Shock Syndrome (TSS): A rare but very serious condition, so don't panic—just change your tampon regularly! **SIX HOURS MAX!**

Unique: What makes you one-of-a-kind. Your quirks, talents, and looks all add up to create YOU, and there's no one else like you in the world!

Urethral Opening/Urethra: The tiny hole where your pee comes out, right below your clitoris. It's not involved in menstruation, but is super important for going to the bathroom.

Uterus: Your baby house! It's the special organ where a baby can grow if you decide to have one later. Each month it prepares for a possible baby, but if there isn't one, it sheds its lining as your period.

Vagina: The stretchy tunnel that connects your outside parts to your uterus, where your period blood comes out, and where babies are born from.

Vulva: The whole outer area of your female private parts, including the labia, clitoris, and the openings to your vagina and urethra.

Wellness: Feeling good in your body, mind, and heart. It's a combination of taking care of your physical health and mental health.

Resources & Interesting Articles

Here are some great articles that I enjoyed reading and got a lot of information from. They could be great Resources for YOU!

Take your time and read through them to see which ones might answer your questions.

♥

7 Amazing Facts about Periods that Everyone Needs to Know – Helping Women period. (2019, April 9). https://www.helpingwomenperiod.org/7-amazing-facts-about-periods-that-everyone-needs-to-know/

11 Signs your Period is Coming: Symptoms & How to Tell. (2024, September 24). Natural Cycles. https://www.naturalcycles.com/cyclematters/signs-your-period-is-coming

All about periods (for teens). (n.d.). https://kidshealth.org/en/teens/menstruation.html

All about puberty (for kids). (n.d.). https://kidshealth.org/en/kids/puberty.html

Brauner, A. M. (2001, August 22). *Period problems: What they mean and when to see the doctor*. WebMD. https://www.webmd.com/women/features/period-problems-what-they-mean-when-to-see-doctor

Department of Health & Human Services. (n.d.). *Puberty*. Better Health Channel. https://www.betterhealth.vic.gov.au/health/healthyliving/puberty

Dove. (n.d.). *The Dove Self-Esteem Project | DOVe*. https://www.dove.com/us/en/dove-self-esteem-project.html?gad_source=1&gbraid=0AAAAADiRVcKsFetkxyFRBX1V7fn0OzrDF&gclid=EAIaIQobChMIodnrpqabiQMVUxitBh0LByFUEAAYASAAEgKu5_D_BwE&gclsrc=aw.ds

Ferguson, S. (2023, February 21). *16 foods to eat (and some to avoid) during your period*. Healthline. https://www.healthline.com/health/womens-health/what-to-eat-during-period

Fletcher, J. (2023, April 25). *What to eat on your period to relieve symptoms*. https://www.medicalnewstoday.com/articles/what-to-eat-on-your-period

Gorvett, Z. (2022, February 24). *How the menstrual cycle changes women's brains – for better*. https://www.bbc.com/future/article/20180806-how-the-menstrual-cycle-changes-womens-brains-every-month

Healthy habits: menstrual hygiene. (2024, May 7). Water, Sanitation, and Environmentally Related Hygiene (WASH). https://www.cdc.gov/hygiene/about/menstrual-hygiene.html

Higuera, V. (2023, April 24). *PMS: Premenstrual syndrome symptoms, treatments, and more*. Healthline. https://www.healthline.com/health/premenstrual-syndrome#symptoms

How Big is a Billion? (n.d.). https://ucmp.berkeley.edu/education/explorations/tours/geotime/guide/billion.html

How to insert non applicator tampon | O.b. FAQ. (n.d.). https://www.ob-tampons.com/faq/how-to-insert-non-applicator-tampon

Irregular periods: When to see a doctor. (n.d.). https://www.unitypoint.org/news-and-articles/irregular-periods-when-to-see-a-doctor

I think I had my first period. How can I be sure? (for teens). (n.d.). https://kidshealth.org/en/teens/expert-period.html

Menstrual cycle: What's normal, what's not. (2023, April 22). Mayo Clinic. https://www.mayoclinic.org/healthy-lifestyle/womens-health/in-depth/menstrual-cycle/art-20047186

Mph, Z. S. (2023, March 29). *What to know about using tampons as a beginner.* https://www.medicalnewstoday.com/articles/how-to-put-in-a-tampon-for-beginners-tampon-types-and-more

NHS inform. (2024, June 7). *Irregular periods.* NHS Inform. https://www.nhsinform.scot/healthy-living/womens-health/girls-and-young-women-puberty-to-around-25/periods-and-menstrual-health/irregular-periods/

Normal menstrual cycle: care instructions. (n.d.). https://myhealth.alberta.ca/Health/aftercareinformation/pages/conditions.aspx?hwid=uh4138

Periods. (2024, May 22). Raising Children Network. https://raisingchildren.net.au/pre-teens/development/periods-hygiene/periods

Physical changes in puberty. (2024, May 22). Raising Children Network. https://raisingchildren.net.au/pre-teens/development/puberty-sexual-development/physical-changes-in-puberty

Practicing Self-Care to feel your best during your period. (n.d.). Self-care During Your Period | Women's Health CT. https://womenshealthct.com/resources-and-faq/resources/practicing-self-care-to-feel-your-best-during-your-period

Premenstrual syndrome (PMS) | Office on Women's Health. (n.d.).

OASH | Office on Women's Health. https://www.womenshealth.gov/menstrual-cycle/premenstrual-syndrome

Puberty Basics (for Teens). (n.d.). https://kidshealth.org/en/teens/puberty.html

Rohatgi, A., & Dash, S. (2023). Period poverty and mental health of menstruators during COVID-19 pandemic: Lessons and implications for the future. *Frontiers in Global Women S Health, 4*. https://doi.org/10.3389/fgwh.2023.1128169

Rosas, K. (2023, June 19). *Menstrual cup folds + tips for getting your cup to open*. Period Nirvana. https://www.periodnirvana.com/menstrual-cup-folds/

Scaccia, A. (2019, April 9). *Everything you need to know about using menstrual cups*. Healthline. https://www.healthline.com/health/womens-health/menstrual-cup

Signs your period is coming. (2022, August 8). WebMD. https://www.webmd.com/women/pms/signs-your-period-is-coming

Tampax. (2021, April 22). *Mood swings during your period and what to do about them*. https://tampax.co.uk/en-gb/period-health/mood-swings-during-your-period/

Tesch, D. (2024, May 24). *13 ways to stop period cramps*. HealthPartners Blog. https://www.healthpartners.com/blog/13-ways-to-stop-period-pain/

The GMC Group. (2021, August 26). *Teen breathe - breathe*. Breathe. https://www.breathemagazine.com/teen-breathe/

The Healthline Editorial Team. (2024, March 27). *6 Home Remedies and OTC Options to Help with Period Cramps*. Healthline. https://www.healthline.com/health/womens-health/menstrual-cramp-remedies

The Royal Women's Hospital. (n.d.). *About your period*. https://www.thewomens.org.au/health-information/periods/periods-overview/about-periods

Toxic shock syndrome - Symptoms & causes - Mayo Clinic. (2022, March 23). Mayo Clinic. https://www.mayoclinic.org/diseases-conditions/toxic-shock-syndrome/symptoms-causes/syc-20355384

Villines, Z. (2023, April 21). *What is menstruation?* https://www.medicalnewstoday.com/articles/154699

Watson, S. (2019, March 8). *How to Deal with Premenstrual Mood Swings.* Healthline. https://www.healthline.com/health/pms-mood-swings

Women's Health Institute. (2023, April 17). *How to feel your best during your period.* Women's Health Institute. https://www.whisanantonio.com/how-to-feel-your-best-during-your-period/

Youtech. (2021, September 28). *How to Embrace Self-Care during your Period.* Women's Health Arizona. https://www.womenshealthaz.com/how-to-embrace-self-care-during-your-period/

Made in the USA
Columbia, SC
21 June 2025

ffd121d8-79cc-4c9f-9684-2abaca7a4c96R01